FLEXIBILITY FOR SPORT

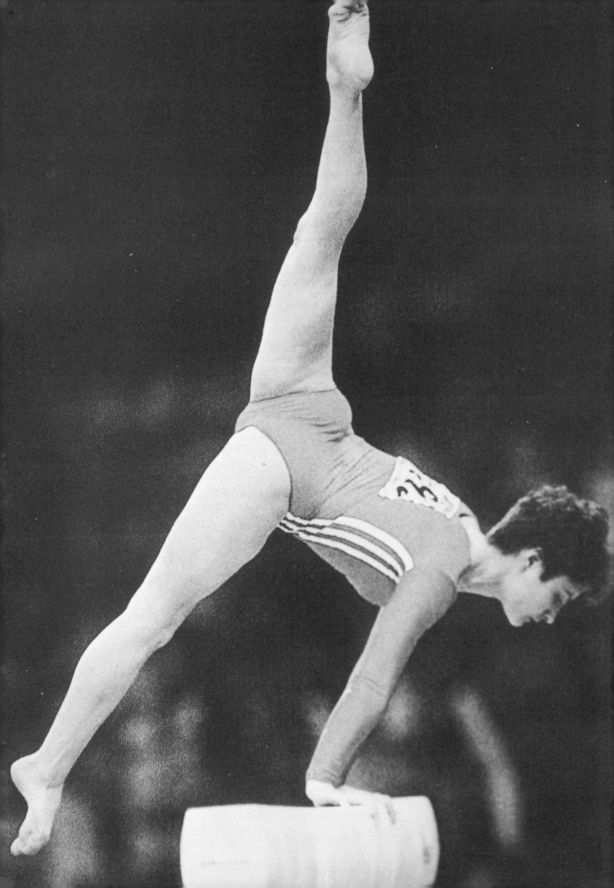

THE • SKILLS • OF • THE • GAME

FLEXIBILITY FOR SPORT

Bob Smith

The Crowood Press

First published in 1994 by
The Crowood Press Ltd
Ramsbury, Marlborough
Wiltshire SN8 2HR

Paperback edition 1996

British Library Cataloguing-in-Publication Data

A catalogue record for this book is available from the British Library.

ISBN 1 85223 985 9

9 9020013
2 3/9/99

Picture Credits
All photographs by Terry Sharpe
Line-drawings by Annette Findlay

Acknowledgements
I should like to thank the following people for providing their time and patience in the compilation of this book: Terry Sharpe for taking the photographs; Jo Prescott, Ben Tan, Julie Lakomy and Mike Waring for being such talented models; Michael Peyrebrune for his modelling and his help with the swimming programme; and special thanks to my wife Sally for her help in the preparation of the final manuscript.

Frontispiece: a gymnast demonstrating excellent range of movement, particularly in the hips and ankles.

Typeset by Avonset, Midsomer Norton, Bath
Printed and bound by J.W. Arrowsmith Limited, Bristol

Contents

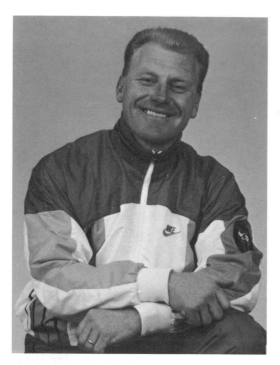

Bob Smith is an accepted authority in the fitness world. He is a full-time lecturer in the Department of Physical Education, Sports Science and Recreation Management at Loughborough University and acts as a consultant for a number of élite performers and training agencies all over the world. He is a member of the Nike Body Élite and in 1992 was the recipient of the Asset Award for Education and the Fitness Professionals' Award of Excellence. He travels the world giving lectures, and holding workshops and seminars as part of his commitment to fitness education. Bob is a competitive triathlete and has represented Great Britain as an age-group competitor.

This is an excellent book on a very important area of a sportsperson's fitness programme. It skilfully and succinctly combines the complicated theory with accurate programme prescription in an easily understandable style. It is essential reading for any athletes, coaches, teachers or exercise professionals who wish to improve their knowledge and be able to apply it in a safe and effective way. The illustrations are first class and clearly show the postures required for safe technique.

Adrian Moorhouse

Flexibility training is now rightly accepted as an important part of fitness preparation. Among sportspeople, however, there is still some misunderstanding and confusion concerning the subject, particularly the question of which are the safest and most effective stretching techniques.

I welcome this book because it deals with the relevant theoretical considerations in a clear and understandable way, as well as fully covering the stretching techniques themselves, including suggestions for specific sports. The book also explains how to include flexibility in the overall training programme.

Bob Smith has considerable expertise and experience in fitness education in general, and flexibility is his speciality. As a lecturer at Loughborough University, responsible for tutoring students on the subject of fitness as well as training teachers of physical education, he is in the forefront of new initiatives, developments and research in his areas of interest. This enables him to be a good practitioner in every sense. This comes through in his book, which makes a valuable contribution to clarifying and informing such an important area of fitness for sport.

Rex Hazeldine
Director, Centre for Coaching and Recreation,
Loughborough University
England Rugby football team Fitness Advisor

Introduction

Flexibility training is rapidly becoming an accepted part of any athlete's regime. Its increase in popularity stems from the awareness that, by increasing a joint's flexibility, the potential of that joint to produce an effective movement pattern in sports performance is significantly enhanced. In addition, it is widely believed that by increasing a joint's flexibility, the potential injury risk to that joint is decreased. With increased flexibility, the muscles, tendons and ligaments around the joint are not put under as much strain in a given movement pattern, as they are when the joint is stiff. This is especially true when an individual is moving through a relatively large range of movement, such as in kicking a ball, or throwing an implement a considerable distance.

It is, of course, also possible to be too flexible, and although this is quite rare in the population as a whole, some people are born with lax ligaments that do not support joints as strongly as they should. Also, some gymnasts and dancers develop extreme ranges of movement, which can cause problems when joints are repeatedly stressed beyond a normal range. Clearly, the key to success in flexibility training is to know how much flexibility is required for a given sport, or simply in daily life, for those keen to be healthier. Balanced flexibility, then, is important for long-term success.

I have used the word athlete throughout this book rather than sportsman/sportswoman/sportsperson in the interests of simplicity. The definition in the *Oxford English Dictionary* of this word is 'competitor or skilled performer in physical exercises; robust or vigorous person'. This seems to be a perfectly apt interpretation.

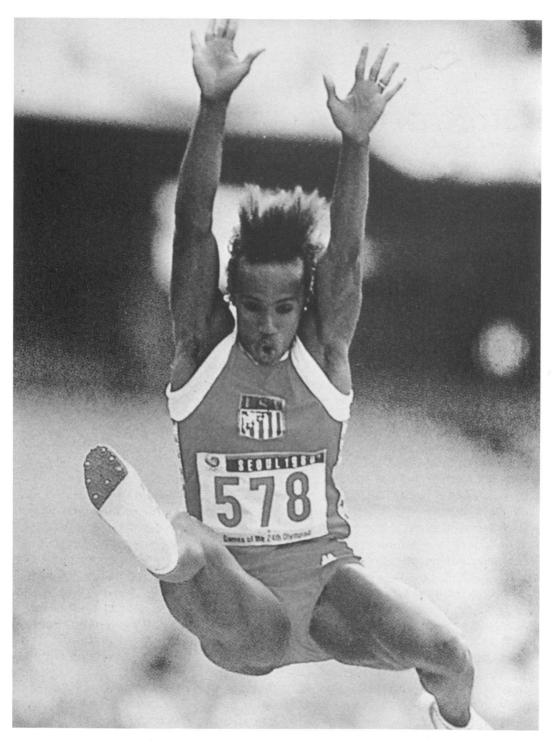

Flexibility demands are not always obvious until a closer examination is taken.

1

Range of Movement

Flexibility is defined as range of movement (ROM), and it is regarded as being joint specific, that is, the ROM in each joint needs to be trained separately; it is perfectly possible, for example, to be very flexible in the hip joint but very inflexible in the shoulder, or to have an excellent ROM in the ankles but be very stiff in the spine. Clearly, a flexibility programme needs to recognize this fact if it is going to be effective. Stretching all the major muscle groups is necessary to achieve a balanced development, which may have an important role to play in the prevention of injury.

Some areas of the body are notoriously stiff in many individuals, and a closer look at these areas proves to be invaluable when concerned with the prescription of stretching exercises. The first problem area is the back of the lower leg (the calf area). Walking and running, especially when the ankle is not used through its full range, may be a contributory factor to this problem, as is the wearing of high-heeled shoes. Such is the structure of the ankle, with a number of muscles converging into the Achilles tendon, that repeated short-range contractions of this musculature appear to have a shortening effect. Regular stretching may, therefore, assist in reducing this problem.

The second problem area is the back of the thigh; trouble here is usually attributable to tight or over-short hamstrings, which affect the posture adversely by pulling down on the pelvis. This causes restricted movement of the pelvis which, in turn, affects the lumbar spine. It is often this postural defect that produces back problems and therefore pain. The other problem with tight hamstrings is that, in any movement that involves flexing the hip (such as kicking, for example), the tightness in the hamstrings will restrict the movement possible to such an extent that they will be severely 'pulled' sooner rather than later in the kicking-action range. Not only will injuries be more likely to occur, but the power of the movement will also be reduced.

The third problem area is the hip region. The area is problematic when considering the development of flexibility owing to the integrated network of ligaments present which ensure joint stability, and the deep socket arrangement of the hip joint. Again, as very stable joints, the hips are not built to provide a wide range of movement like the shoulder, and so developing a wide range of movement in this area is both difficult and affected by age. It appears that greater ranges of hip flexibility are only possible before the age of about ten years, after which the increased tightness in the ligaments makes extreme ranges of hip flexibility, as displayed in

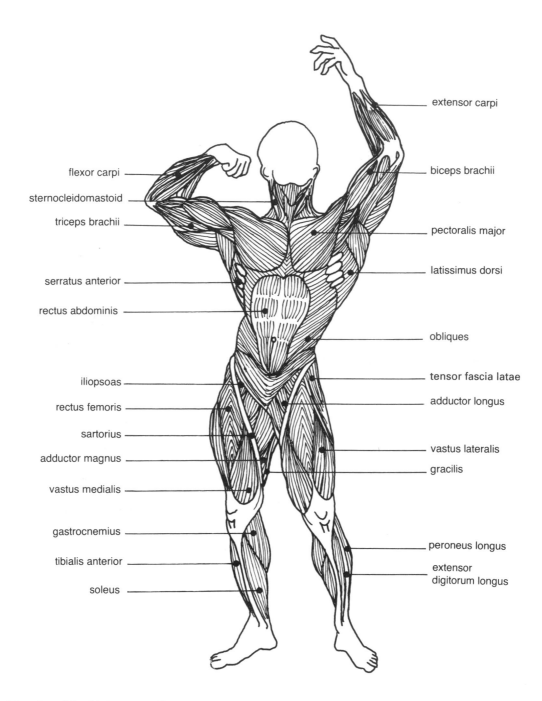

extensor carpi

flexor carpi

biceps brachii

sternocleidomastoid

triceps brachii

pectoralis major

latissimus dorsi

serratus anterior

rectus abdominis

obliques

iliopsoas

tensor fascia latae

rectus femoris

adductor longus

sartorius

adductor magnus

vastus lateralis

gracilis

vastus medialis

gastrocnemius

tibialis anterior

peroneus longus

extensor
digitorum longus

soleus

Figs 1 and 2   Major superficial muscle groups.

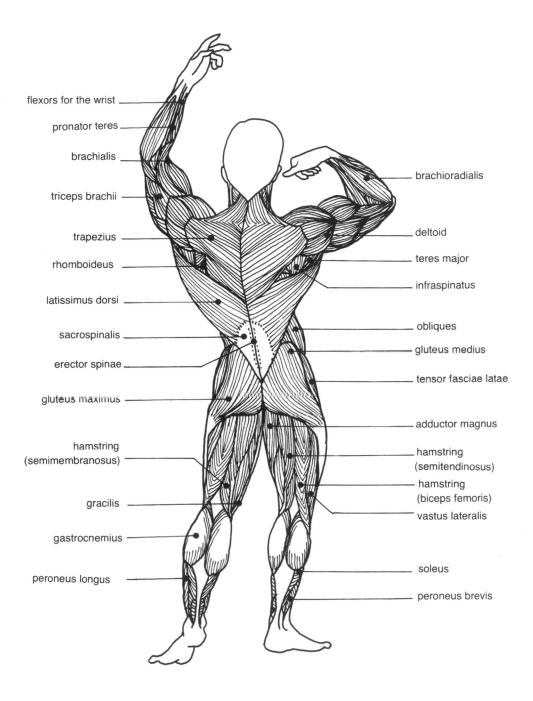

flexors for the wrist

pronator teres

brachialis

triceps brachii

trapezius

rhomboideus

latissimus dorsi

sacrospinalis

erector spinae

gluteus maximus

hamstring
(semimembranosus)

gracilis

gastrocnemius

peroneus longus

brachioradialis

deltoid

teres major

infraspinatus

obliques

gluteus medius

tensor fasciae latae

adductor magnus

hamstring
(semitendinosus)

hamstring
(biceps femoris)

vastus lateralis

soleus

peroneus brevis

Fig 2.

the splits position for example, very difficult to achieve, and perfect positions nearly impossible.

The ligaments which are responsible for the increased tightness and stability in the hip area are the pubofemoral ligament, the iliofemoral ligament, the ischiofemoral ligament and the transverse acetabular ligament. Their united

efforts tend to restrict, rather than promote range of motion, and therefore their influence should be taken into account when considering stretching exercises for this area.

The lower back is the fourth problem area, and tightness here is often caused by inactivity, too much sitting in chairs or the wearing of high-heeled shoes.

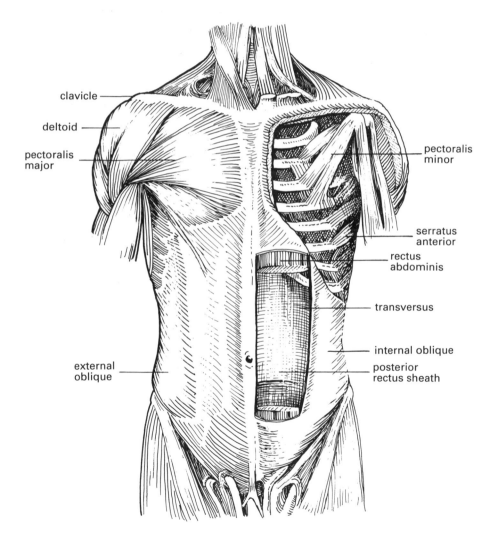

Fig 3 Musculature of the chest and abdomen.

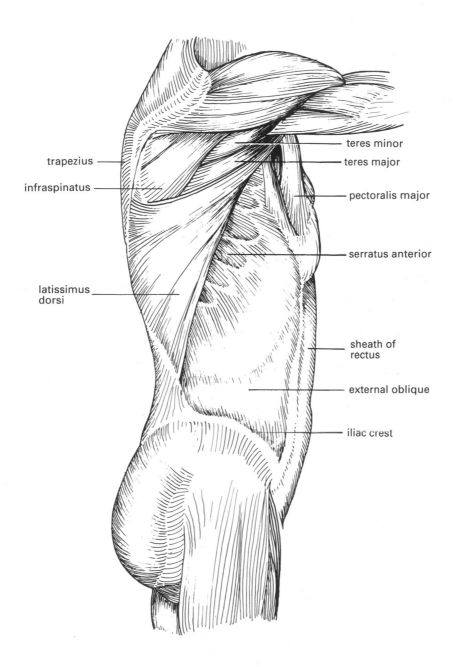

Fig 4   Lateral musculature of the chest and abdomen.

Restricted movement in the lower back makes flexion (bending) difficult, and this has a knock-on effect for other areas of the body. There is usually a close tie-in between tight lower-back muscles and tight hamstrings and hip flexor muscles. This is because of the integrated structure of the hips, the pelvis and the lumbar spine.

The chest is the fifth problem area, especially in individuals who do weight training. The tendency is to perform many exercises for the chest itself rather than for the opposing muscles of the upper back and back of the shoulder, especially the rhomboid, trapezius 3 and posterior deltoid muscles. The result of inadequate compensatory stretching of this area is a tight chest musculature, which can lead to a round-shouldered posture on the one hand, and when weight training, a greater tendency to over-stretch the short chest muscles, especially pectoralis major and minor, on the other. Additionally, shortness in the anterior deltoid and the short head of the biceps muscle as it originates on the coracoid (front point) of the shoulder, can lead to these muscles being over-stretched in weight-training exercises such as dumb-bell flyes, bench press and pec-dec movements. To avoid these potential problems, a balanced weight-training routine, coupled with regular stretching, should form the basis of an individual's programme.

TERMINOLOGY

In some quarters, *flexibility* is used synonymously with *mobility* and *suppleness*. However, I will distinguish between the three. *Mobility* refers to

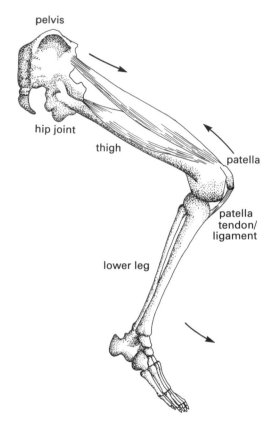

Fig 5 Range of movement in a synovial joint (the knee joint).

movements in the inner and middle ranges of a joint (*see* fig 5). These movements are very usefully performed in a warm-up as they increase the temperature of the structures around the joint, especially of a substance called synovial fluid, which is responsible for joint lubrication. It effectively acts like the oil in a car engine, in that it lubricates, protects and promotes the smooth running of the parts of the joint. The surfaces that come together in a joint and are bathed in synovial fluid are known as the articular surfaces.

14

When the structures around the joint become warm and receive a greater blood supply, they become more pliable. The joint's viscosity (resistance to movement) is decreased and this enhances the overall ROM by taking away some of the limitation to it.

Mobility, then, is a component of ROM, but is not synonymous with it, as it does not refer to all components in this context. Similarly, another component of ROM is *suppleness*. This refers to the pliability, or stretchability, of muscle and connective tissue. The more supple the muscle, the less resistance there will be to limit ROM. A useful way to distinguish, therefore, between flexibility and suppleness is to state that we have flexible joints and supple muscles. Joints display a range of movement (flexibility), but muscles play a role in contributing to the range of movement, which can be either positive (supple muscles) or negative (unsupple muscles).

Researchers have shown that, in terms of resistance to ROM, it is the suppleness of the muscles and their connective tissue that represents the biggest changeable factor when wanting to improve flexibility. Other factors – for example, the shape of the joint or its anatomical make-up – are not changeable without damaging the joint, unless a person is born with a particular condition commonly known as lax ligaments. However, through stretching muscle and connective tissue, large increases in ROM can be achieved naturally.

Stretching, therefore, is the means by which we improve our *flexibility* most, and as such should be included in everyone's daily routine, be they athletes or fitness-conscious individuals. We automatically become less flexible as we get older; the only way to slow down this natural ageing process is to stretch on a regular basis.

Many models of fitness have been suggested to cover all possible factors that an athlete might need to include in a programme. Table 1 (overleaf) gives an example of such a model, showing how flexibility can be a component of all fitness programmes.

Following on from Table 1, Table 1a indicates some of the ways in which flexibility training can be used within the overall programme. An explanation of the methods of stretching indicated here will follow, but first, it is necessary to explain the important principles underlying flexibility training; in this way a fuller technical understanding can be obtained as well as a clearer indication of its importance in the 'fitness model' of any athlete.

I will tackle this from two angles: from the structural angle – which covers factors concerning muscle, bone and connective tissue – and from the neurological angle, which deals with the role of the controlling mechanisms of the brain and the neurological pathways.

STRUCTURAL FACTORS

Joints

Because flexibility is joint specific, a knowledge of the important joints, as far as participation in sports is concerned, is essential. Joint specificity is a very important concept and means that a person's flexibility cannot be established by any one measurement. Not only does an individual's ROM vary between one joint and the next, but it will also vary

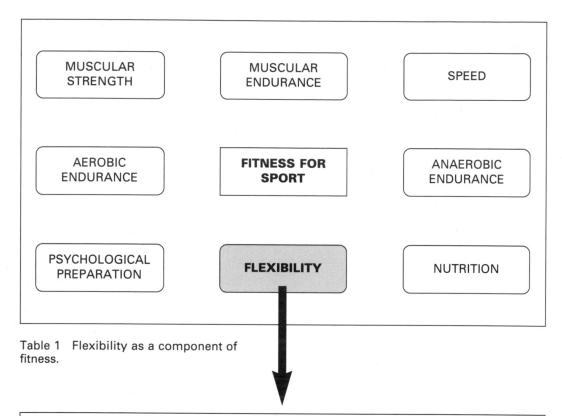

Table 1   Flexibility as a component of fitness.

Type	Purpose
Personal Stretching Short Hold	As part of a Warm-up Preparation Stretches
Personal Stretching Long Hold	As part of a Cool-Down for Recovery and Development of ROM
Partner Stretching Long Hold	Further Development of ROM
PNF Stretches Personal and Partner	Further Development of ROM

Table 1a   Uses of flexibility training.

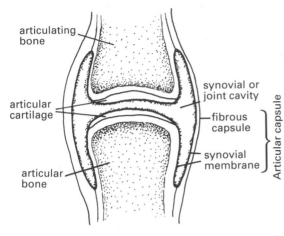

Fig 6 A typical synovial joint.

from one movement to the next. For example, in the shoulder joint there will be a range of flexion, a separate range of extension, a yet different range of abduction and adduction, and so on (*see* table 2).

Joints which produce movements are collectively known as *synovial joints* because they all share a similar structure (*see* fig 6). Synovial joints are freely movable and are made up of two bones coming together (articular surfaces). The ends of the bones are protected by articular cartilage, which is bathed in synovial fluid, a form of lymph that comes from the synovial membrane. Ligaments hold the bones together and provide stability, while muscles and their tendons facilitate the movement of the joint.

Not all synovial joints perform the same movements, as this is determined to a large extent by the structure of the joint. Table 2 (overleaf) indicates the most important synovial joints in the body, their movement potential, and their classification. By studying this

table, important information about the movements required to produce stretches can be learned. Every joint has the potential for a certain range of movement; knowing what these are will help the athlete devise a fuller stretching regime.

It is important to remember that, in terms of flexibility training, an individual will have a range of movement in all the possible options listed in the centre column of table 2. Sometimes the term *hyper* is used with flexion and extension movements to indicate that a person has an excellent ROM. Hyperflexion of the shoulder joint, for example, would indicate that the movement is taken beyond the normal range of flexion; this would be an essential prerequisite for a swimmer or a gymnast (*see* fig 7).

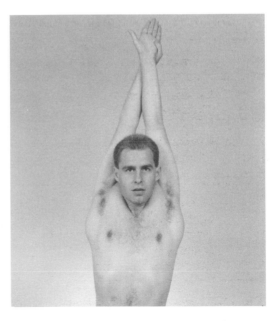

Fig 7 Hyperflexion of the shoulder. A swimmer showing excellent ROM.

Body Part	Movements Possible	Joint Classification
Shoulder Joint	Flexion, extension, abduction, adduction, circumduction, rotation	BALL AND SOCKET
Scapula	Abduction, adduction, elevation, depression, rotation	GLIDING (Clavicle and scapula)
Hip	Flexion, extension, abduction, adduction, circumduction, rotation	BALL AND SOCKET
Spine	Flexion, extension, lateral flexion and extension, rotation	MAINLY GLIDING (Not all areas of the spine can perform all these movements)
Elbow	Flexion, extension	HINGE
Radio-Ulna	Pronation, supination	PIVOT
Wrist	Flexion, extension, abduction, adduction, circumduction	CONDYLOID
Knee	Flexion, extension, slight medial and lateral rotation	COMPLEX HINGE
Ankle	Flexion, extension	HINGE
Foot (Mid-tarsals)	Inversion, eversion, abduction, adduction	GLIDING

Table 2   Joints and their potential for movement.

MOVEMENTS

The following examples exactly illustrate the movements in the centre column of table 2: when one of these movements is performed and held at the end of the range, it will elicit a stretch in the appropriate muscles.

Fig 8   Movements of the body.

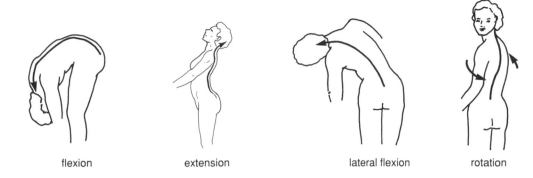

| flexion | extension | lateral flexion | rotation |

Fig 8a   Movements of the spinal column.

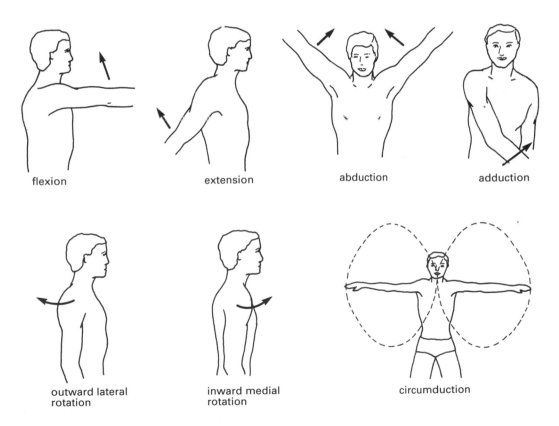

| flexion | extension | abduction | adduction |

| outward lateral rotation | inward medial rotation | circumduction |

Fig 8b   Movements of the shoulder joint.

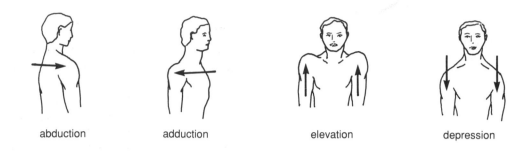

Fig 8c   Movements of the shoulder girdle.

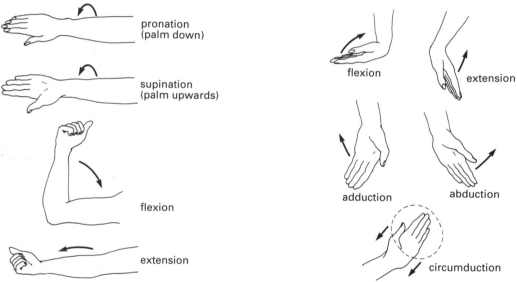

Fig 8d   Movements of the elbow joint.   Fig 8e   Movements of the wrist joint.

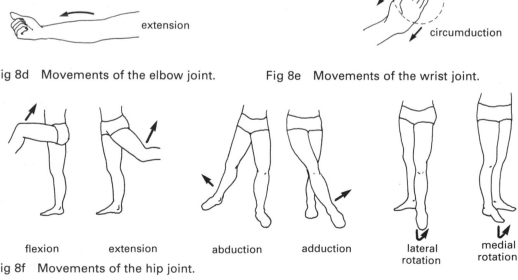

Fig 8f   Movements of the hip joint.

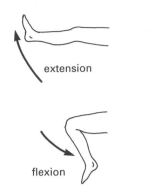

extension

flexion

Fig 8g   Movements of the knee joint.

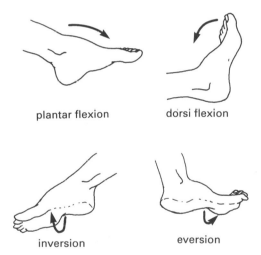

plantar flexion

dorsi flexion

inversion

eversion

Fig 8h   Movements of the ankle joint.

Muscles and Tendons

In terms of improving ROM, the level of resistance in muscles and connective tissue is the biggest single changeable factor. An understanding, therefore, of how muscles and tendons are made up will be an important first step in deciding on the best way to go about decreasing the resistance they provide when trying to achieve a particular range of movement.

Muscles either attach directly to bone, or are attached via a tendon. Tendons are fairly rigid structures made up almost entirely of a protein called collagen. Collagen has an amazing tensile strength but is not very elastic, therefore tendons do not stretch a great deal, nor should the athlete try to stretch them specifically. Over-stretching a tendon can cause injury, which can often be prolonged because the relatively poor blood supply to the tendon makes the repair process slow. Collagen is also present within the muscle unit acting as a connective tissue between muscle fibres and bundles of muscle fibres. Fig 9 shows the make-up of a muscle and its connective tissue.

Fig 9 also shows how sarcomeres make up myofibrils, which in turn make up muscle fibres. Each muscle fibre is surrounded by a layer of connective tissue called the *endomysium*. Muscle fibres are arranged in bundles called *fasciculi* and each fasciculus is surrounded by connective tissue called the *perimysium*. Bundles of fibres are also bound together to form the whole muscle unit, and these are surrounded by a superficial layer of connective tissue called the *epimysium*. The sheer amount of connective tissue within a muscle unit gives an indication of the importance of con-

21

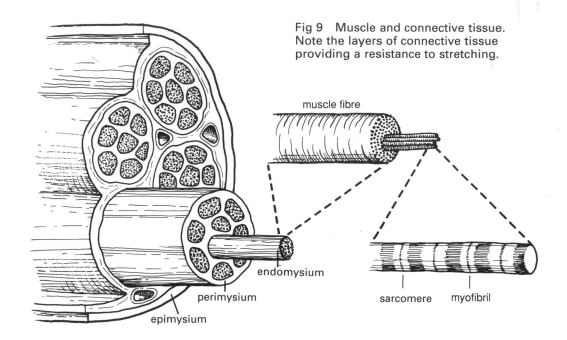

Fig 9   Muscle and connective tissue. Note the layers of connective tissue providing a resistance to stretching.

muscle fibre

endomysium

perimysium

epimysium

sarcomere   myofibril

nective tissue to stretching. It adds strength and resilience to a muscle and is certainly a part to be taken seriously.

The functional, contractile part of a muscle is the sarcomere. Within the sarcomere, the proteins actin and myosin are pulled across one another to develop tension in a muscle. This tension is referred to as a *contraction*, and is achieved when structures called cross-bridges cause the protein filaments to slide across one another. This *sliding filament theory* of muscle contraction is currently the most plausible explanation of how this process works.

The muscle is thus able to contract and, as the protein filaments return to their original positions, relax; and when pulled apart, stretch. These proteins always return to their original length when the work is done, much like a rubber band. Consequently, it is thought

that the muscle itself presents little resistance to ROM. It appears that it has plenty of lengthening potential before it reaches its critical limit and tears. It is rather the connective tissue that lies around the muscle fibres and around the bundles of muscle fibres (the fasciculi) that is the principal cause of the resistance to stretch.

Depending on the particular make-up of the three layers of connective tissue, there may be a great deal of resistance to stretching the muscle unit, or not very much. Another important connective tissue, along with collagen, is *elastin*, which is much more pliable, and consequently much more responsive to stretching. The proportion of elastin to collagen, therefore, may be an important genetic factor influencing ROM. It does appear that some people are more supple quite naturally, even though they may be sedentary and do little or no stretching.

MUSCLE PAIRS

Muscles can be thought of as working in pairs around any one joint. That is, as one muscle (or group of muscles) contracts to produce a movement, its opposite must relax to allow that movement to take place. For example, when the elbow is flexed by the biceps muscle contracting, the triceps muscle relaxes. As the biceps achieves full (peak) contraction, the triceps has to elongate to accommodate this position. We refer to this elongation as stretching. Further, it can be thought of as *active stretching* because the proportion of stretch in the triceps is determined by the degree of contraction in the biceps. The action of one muscle contracting determines the degree of stretch in its opposite muscle.

This process of one muscle contracting and its opposite relaxing occurs in all joints around the body, with only a few paradoxical exceptions. The complete process is known as *reciprocal innervation*, or *reciprocal inhibition*. One muscle is innervated to contract, and its opposite is inhibited so that it relaxes. By being relaxed it puts up less resistance, of course, to the process of stretching.

We refer to the contracting muscle as the *prime mover* or *agonist*, and the relaxing muscle as the *antagonist*. Thus, for example, when the hamstrings contract (agonists), the quadriceps relax (antagonists). But when the quadriceps contract, *they* become the agonists and the hamstrings relax, becoming the antagonists. Clearly this is a reciprocal, or interchangeable arrangement, whereby muscles play different roles at different times.

We can now see the importance of suppleness more clearly, as a contributory factor to ROM. The suppleness of the antagonist muscle in any joint movement will enhance the movement potential. Similarly, a lack of suppleness will inhibit range of movement and may put the muscle and connective tissue under considerable strain.

The antagonist muscle in a joint movement can also be stretched without relying on the force of the contraction of the agonist. In this case the stretch is said to be *passive*. If a hand, gravity or a partner is used to help stretch the hamstrings, for example, all these aids would produce passive stretching of the hamstrings; as we shall see, they also represent effective ways of increasing ROM by stretching the antagonist muscle (*see* figs 10a and b).

NEUROLOGICAL FACTORS

The process by which muscles contract or relax, and the sophisticated interrelationship between muscles undertaking specific roles, is under the control of the central nervous system. This control mechanism is referred to as neurological control, a basic understanding of which is essential if effective development of flexibility is to be undertaken.

There are two aspects of neurological control that are of major importance to flexibility training: the *myotatic stretch reflex*, and the *golgi-tendon organ reflex* (GTO), or *inverse stretch reflex*.

Myotatic Stretch Reflex

Whenever a muscle is quickly stretched, the muscle spindles that control the

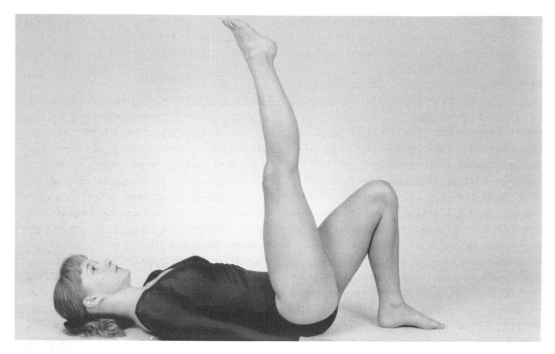

Fig 10a   Active stretching of the hamstring.

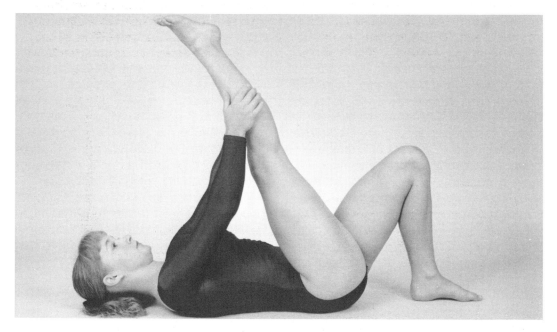

Fig 10b   Passive stretching of the hamstring.

24

stimulation of that muscle react by initiating a reflex contraction. This is to prevent over-stretching (*see* fig 11). The result of the myotatic reflex springing into action is a contraction of the muscle that is being stretched. Although this may seem paradoxical, it is worth remembering that this is a protective mechanism to prevent damage to the muscle from over-stretching.

One important practical application of this knowledge is that, if a muscle is to be stretched effectively, the myotatic reflex must be overcome or *desensitized*. This is usually achieved when a more stable environment in the muscle exists, so moving slowly into stretch positions, and then holding the position, will minimise the stretch reflex in the first instance, and allow relaxation of the muscle spindles once the stretch is held. This allows the muscle and connective tissue to stretch with reduced resistance from this neurological process. This form of stretching is known as *static stretching* and is referred to in fig 10a

and b; it will be explained more fully later (*see* page 34).

Golgi-Tendon Organs

GTOs are also a protective mechanism, but these receptors are situated in the tendons, at the junction of the muscle and tendon. Their role is to monitor changes in tension inside the muscle. If the tension inside the muscle achieves a certain critical level, the GTOs respond by sending a message to the spinal cord (called the afferent message). Then, an efferent message is sent back to the muscle spindles causing them to be inhibited so that they have to relax. This is a reflex action which is not under conscious control.

When this process occurs, and the GTOs fire in this way, the muscle relaxes more than normal, and greater stretching can be achieved. Because tension in the muscle manifests itself by pulling the tendon (which is what the GTOs sense), the GTOs can detect a strong stretch, as

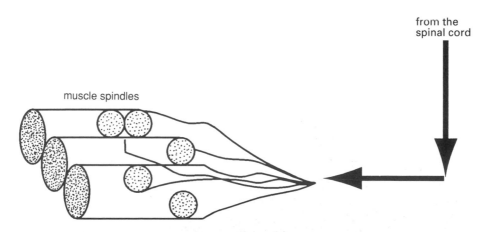

Fig 11   Muscle spindles and their control mechanism via the spinal cord. The myotatic reflex is a reflex mechanism involving these spindles, which causes the muscle to contract when quickly stretched.

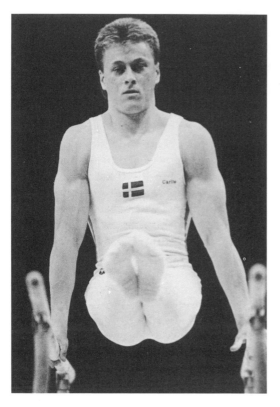

Good flexibility results in less wasted energy when it matters.

well as a contraction. They both pull on the tendon. However, it is much more difficult to obtain a sufficiently large amount of tension to cause the GTOs to fire through conventional stretching, so a contraction of the muscle about to be stretched is used to serve this purpose. This explains why it is thought that you gain greater relaxation in muscles, and hence increased stretch, when a muscle is contracted immediately before it is stretched.

In simple terms, then, when a muscle is placed in a stretched position, and is then contracted, enough tension is created for the GTOs to fire. This firing will result in the immediate reflex relaxation of that muscle. Contraction-relaxation techniques are therefore used because they trigger the GTO mechanism, and ultimately achieve a greater stretch response. These techniques will be described in detail shortly, but many of them come under the general heading of PNF techniques referred to in figs 14a and b. PNF stands for *proprioceptive neuromuscular facilitation*.

2
Factors Affecting Flexibility

Before moving on to the techniques for improving or maintaining range of movement, I will discuss some miscellaneous factors that may affect flexibility. Some factors you are born with, like gender and body type (somatotype), and others are related to natural development such as ageing. A third factor, of course, is training (stretching) itself, which will affect to some degree the influence of these miscellaneous factors on the body.

GENDER DIFFERENCES

Although most people would agree that males are less flexible than females, there is, in fact, a lack of conclusive evidence to support this statement. However, there appear to be several anatomical differences between males and females that give females an advantage when displaying ROM, and I will turn to these now.

Because of the different shape of the female pelvis, which is designed to be wider and flatter than the male's, there is greater potential for flexibility. The female's lighter bone structure is another advantage. During pregnancy a woman experiences greater potential for ROM owing to the increased secretion of the hormone relaxin, which, as the name suggests, has a relaxing effect on the ligamentous structures, especially around the pelvis. It may also be that during the course of a woman's daily life, the differing hormone levels of oestrogen and progesterone also play a part in affecting ROM, but no conclusive data is as yet available on this issue.

On the other side of the coin, there is nothing inherently wrong with the male body that makes it naturally less flexible. Various hypotheses have been put forward to suggest why males tend not to be as flexible, and such issues as lifestyle, exercise patterns and activity preferences have been considered. However, all have failed to explain fully any gender differences. Observing a male ice skater, diver, gymnast or swimmer tends to dispel the belief that males cannot possess a complete range of movement in all joint complexes, if indeed this was ever seriously in question.

Somatotype and Flexibility

Studies that have addressed this issue have been largely inconclusive, so that it seems no one body type is naturally more flexible than another. Investigations into the effect of body-weight, height, body fat and lean muscle tissue have all ended with inconclusive findings. The net result is that both fat and lean people can be either flexible or inflexible. Similarly, muscular people are at no more of a disadvantage in terms of ROM than thin, non-muscular people.

The latter point may come as a surprise to some readers who have heard talk of *muscle boundness* that occurs in people who lift heavy weights. In fact, restricted range of motion in joints has been seen in patients who, for one reason or another, have had a limb immobilized for a period of time. One might infer, therefore, that restriction to joint flexibility may be the result of poor weight-training practice rather than the undertaking of weight training itself. Short-range or restricted-range movements are the worst culprits.

Studies in the 1970s and 1980s revealed that weight-training exercises performed slowly through a full range of movement actually improved flexibility. The success was in part attributable to the enhanced reciprocal inhibition (just described) which is produced by one muscle contracting fully, eliciting relaxation and stretch in the antagonist.

What does appear to be confirmed with regard to body types is that flexibility is specific to each joint and additionally to each movement within each joint. Also, it is the practice of performing flexibility-enhancing movements that promotes ROM, rather than other factors that are subject to many uncontrollable variables.

The process of stretching helps reduce the viscosity in muscle as I have mentioned, and this is an important factor; viscosity, to a large extent, is the result of inelastic connective tissue, especially collagen, and appears to increase with age regardless of gender or body type.

Age and Flexibility

It seems quite clear that we get less flexible as we get older, and that the only way to combat the ageing process is to be active, both in joint mobility exercise and in stretching the muscles and connective tissues. However, there appear to be critical periods of flexibility development, of which the coaches of aspiring youngsters should be aware if these periods are to be used to their full advantage.

Research suggests that youngsters are very supple and that this is a major determinant of overall ROM. After an initial levelling off of flexibility in the first three years of life, improvements in ROM are again seen in the formative (primary school) years. It appears that a prime time to improve flexibility, from a training point of view, is between the ages of seven and eleven. After that there is another plateau period before a decline sets in during adolescence. Following adolescence there is a steady decline throughout the rest of adult life.

In simple terms then, if aspiring athletes can be encouraged to develop their flexibility in their primary school years, they can literally be setting themselves up for life. However, a note of caution should be struck when considering a stretching programme for a young performer. During periods of rapid development and growth, the youngster is at risk from both over-use injury and acute traumatic injury from insensitive practice. Bones, ligaments, tendons and muscles are all susceptible to injury during the formative years, and while, perhaps, insensitive strength training is more of a risk because it can include the use of relatively heavy

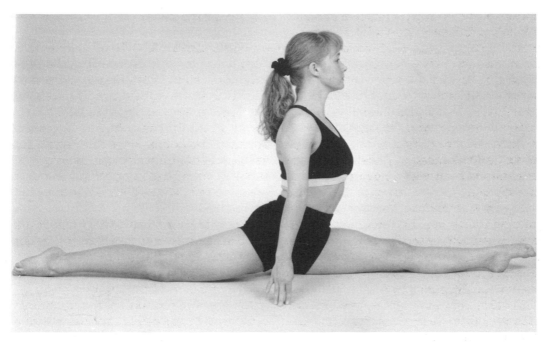

Fig 12   Excellent range of movement.

Care should be taken when devising.

resistance, flexibility training also needs careful consideration.

Over-stretching tissues that are undergoing development, especially ligaments, can be a major concern, as can the forcing of joints beyond their normal range. This can produce joint laxity. Chapter 4 on 'Stretches to Avoid' should provide a useful starting point for weeding out some of the most severely criticized movements in this regard, but coaches and trainers in sports where the demands on flexibility are great, might be tempted to take short cuts by using more violent stretching techniques. I would strongly advise against this because of the potential long-term damage that may result.

There is no substitute for a carefully structured programme that is gradual and progressive and that uses safe and effective techniques. This is also important when a stretching programme is being devised for the elderly, especially elderly women who appear to be at greater risk of bone damage after the menopause. Bone softening, a condition known as osteoporosis or porous bone, has been termed the silent thief because of the debilitating effect it has on bone density. Insensitive postures or violent movements that stress bones and joints may hinder rather than promote the healthy development of the skeleton.

Another cause for concern that develops with age is the increased presence of the connective tissue collagen, mentioned earlier. Collagen's strength appears to be the product of a rope-like, triple-helix arrangement, in structural terms, and a strong biochemical make-up combining proline, glycine and

29

hydroxyproline in a polypeptide chain. Put simply, this means that collagen has exceptional structural and biochemical strength combined with very limited elasticity. As such, it is a major limiting factor to flexibility, especially, but not exclusively, in older people.

By following the stretches in the 'Long-Hold Stretches' and 'Short-Hold Stretches' sections in Chapter 5, paying particular attention to the safety guidelines, there is no reason why both young and old, both élite and novice, cannot develop their flexibility. The younger the person when commencing the programme, the greater will be the potential gain, and I would encourage all parents and coaches to spend time on flexibility training using the developmental programmes suggested later in the text. *Everyone* can improve their flexibility; how great the improvement will be is influenced by many factors, the most important of which I have discussed in this chapter.

STRENGTH TRAINING

It is important at this point to say a word about strength training in relation to the development of flexibility. Ideally, strong, supple muscles are required in sporting activities so that the joints can perform their tasks effectively, while at the same time protecting themselves. Also, if the muscle contracting to move the joint (the agonist) lacks strength, a deficiency in active flexibility may result. Kicking a ball or swinging a golf club, for example, require a reasonable amount of active flexibility, which will be achieved by the strength of one muscle and the suppleness of its opposite, in combination.

Strength training, therefore, can be seen to be important in the development of ROM, and must not be overlooked. However, depending on the age, fitness level and aspiration of the individual concerned, the type of strength training used will vary. Some individuals may want strength but not the bulk associated with very heavy resistance work. A marathon runner, for example, requires enough strength combined with speed to perform well in a marathon, but does not want a heavy body to carry around the course. It is well established that an increase in muscle mass increases the overall weight of the individual, which can be counterproductive in some sports.

Others, for example swimmers, will require a balance between upper- and lower-body strength. If the legs are very heavy owing to a large muscle mass, they may give added drag and impede the speed of the swimmer. Similarly, gymnasts require functional strength. They need a favourable strength-to-body-weight ratio, and like runners do not want to be too heavy.

The development of strength, given all these factors, will need to be specific, both to the joints important to the particular sport, and to the requirements of the sport itself, once a firm base is developed from which to proceed. Some individuals will need to use only body-weight as a resistance to build strength, others will require the use of pulleys and rubber tubing (swimmers, for example), and still others will use machines and free-weights in various combinations to achieve their specific requirements.

Whatever the type of weight training, if controlled, full-range movements are performed, flexibility can be enhanced at the

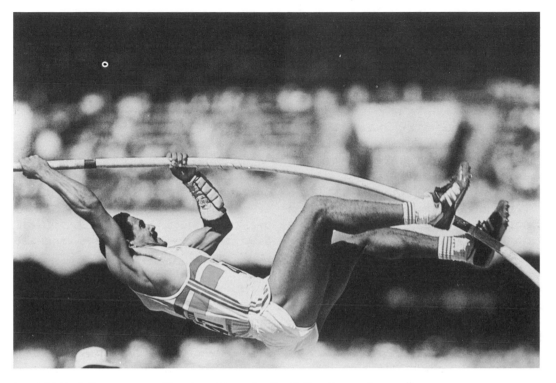

In multidisciplinary sports like decathlon, the flexibility demands are diverse and complex. Notice the potential for strain on the shoulders.

same time as strength. This will be both safer and more effective in the long term than other, gimmicky techniques that employ short-range pulsing-type movements, which may lead to muscle shortening rather than muscle suppleness. Good posture when performing exercises, as well as isolation of the movements required, are also important safety factors.

Safety factors are especially important when dealing with youngsters. Strength-training techniques, as well as flexibility techniques, need to be taught carefully, thoroughly and knowledgeably by trained individuals. The dangers of excessive or violent exercise to the young skeleton are well documented; these are of special concern in periods of rapid growth when temporary imbalances may occur in bone, muscle and connective tissue development. Clearly, insensitive practice at these critical stages of development has the potential to be severely debilitating.

31

3
Stretching Techniques

Having identified some of the key theoretical aspects of flexibility training, I will now consider how to apply these principles to create safe and effective strategies to improve flexibility. In doing so there are a number of stretching techniques available to the athlete, which could be incorporated into a flexibility training programme.

PERSONAL STRETCHING

This form of stretching is obviously performed alone and can be one of two basic types: *active* or *passive*.

Active Stretching

This form of stretching is useful in a sport-specific context, and involves controlled replication of the movement patterns in a particular sport, to reflect accurately both the range of movement in that sport, and the specific movement pattern. Because the amount of stretch in one muscle (the antagonist) is determined by the force of the contraction in the other muscle (the agonist), this form of stretching has the advantage of developing both strength and suppleness around a joint. Active stretching can be both static and ballistic/dynamic.

An example of the static version occurs when a gymnast stands on one leg and lifts the other so that the foot is next to the ear. This posture shows excellent flexibility, but is only possible because of the strength of the hip flexors that hold this static position, and the suppleness of the hamstrings and adductors that allow this freedom of movement. A split leap, on the other hand, is a much more dynamic movement, and is an example of active ballistic stretching (*see* fig 13).

Ballistic Stretching

This form of stretching involves the active movements of a limb, usually at speed, in an attempt to increase ROM. It takes the form either of repetitive bouncing-type movements, or swinging movements. However, ballistic stretching has received severe criticism in recent years, for three main reasons:

1. It works against the protective mechanism of the myotatic stretch reflex. As the muscle is quickly stretched its automatic reaction is for the muscle to *contract*. This conflict within the muscle is thought to be potentially dangerous, in that the performer is attempting to stretch the muscle while the central nervous system is sending a signal for it to contract.

2. Research into this form of stretching,

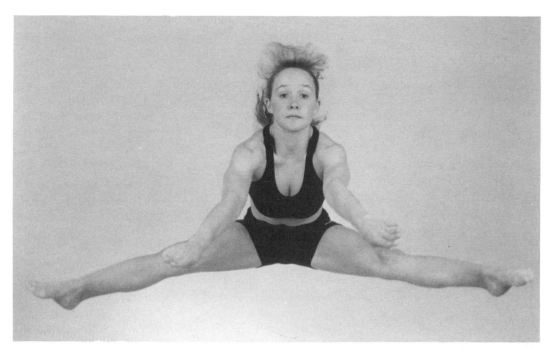

Fig 13   A split leap showing active dynamic flexibility

although not extensive, has tended to indicate that the muscle is the structure most affected by using this technique. As I have mentioned already, the muscle does not appear to be the major factor in limiting flexibility, and so the increased cost of performing ballistic stretching may outweigh the benefit of targeting a structure which already has a good deal of natural elasticity. The connective tissue in muscle appears to give much greater resistance to ROM, so will yield greater gains if properly stretched by static means.

3. The potential for damage is great owing to the speed with which the limb arrives at the end of the range. Momentum may allow the limb to go beyond a safe range and consequently the joint structures, especially the liga-ments, will take the strain. The muscle is also likely to be over-stretched beyond its critical limit because of the speed of the action. This is particularly relevant in structures like the spine, where a good deal of damage can be done easily. In this regard, care must also be taken with flexibility tests that attempt to evaluate dynamic flexibility. Spinal twisting movements, in particular, can be very dangerous.

It is for these reasons that I would not recommend ballistic stretching as a technique to improve flexibility. Active movements may be used in practising a sport performance, but not exclusively for developing flexibility (*see also* Chapter 4 on 'Stretches to Avoid').

33

Static Stretching

This is widely believed to be one of the safest techniques, and should be used extensively by all athletes. There are two ways in which static stretching can be used effectively in a sporting pro-gramme. These will be referred to as *short hold* and *long hold*. Both tech-niques are passive in that gravity, or another part of the body (usually a hand) produces the stretch rather than the muscular contraction of the agonist, or momentum.

SHORT-HOLD STRETCHING

Static stretches which are held for 8–10 seconds can be useful in the preparation for, and recovery from, exercise. The aim of this kind of stretching is to prepare muscles for the activity to follow on the one hand, and to help in the cool-down process on the other.

After a period of 5–8 minutes of movements that gently increase the temperature of the body and of in-dividual muscles, short-hold stretches can be used to promote further relaxa-tion of the muscle spindles and some elongation of muscle and connective tissue. The benefit of this is to ensure that joints have experienced an in-creased range, in a controlled situation, before more vigorous activity places them in a more challenging situation.

After exercise, a training session or a game, a degree of muscle shortening will have occurred as a natural con-sequence of repeated contractions of the muscles. Short-hold stretching can then be used literally to stretch out and relax the structures. This technique is parti-cularly useful for individuals new to stretching, or for those who previously have not bothered to stretch. Repeating the warm-up stretches will facilitate a more complete cool-down and hopefully promote the well-being of the joints.

Work in the 1960s suggested that stretching after exercise reduces or even prevents post-exercise soreness (*see* Chapter 8). However, recent evidence seems to suggest that this is not the case, and no amount of stretching of any kind can actually help if a muscle has been sufficiently damaged. The secret to avoiding or minimizing soreness is to increase the intensity of exercise gradually over a period of time, and to use techniques that do not work against the body's natural potential. Any unaccustomed activity is likely to create post-exercise soreness, which is often referred to as DOMS (delayed onset muscle soreness).

LONG-HOLD STRETCHING

Short-hold stretching used after exercise can be of value as stated above, but long-hold stretches will definitely be better. Long-hold static stretching should therefore be used whenever pos-sible as part of the cool-down procedure after training and competition, and for specific training sessions aimed at de-veloping flexibility. Gymnasts, dancers and swimmers, for example, will also use long-hold stretching in their warm-up preparation owing to the increased demand their sports place on range of movement.

I have identified lack of suppleness in the muscle as a major limiting factor to ROM, and established that suppleness is mainly affected by connective tissue in muscle and tendons. The emphasis should, therefore, be placed on the muscle and its connective tissue, and extreme caution taken with tendons. It is worth reiterating that they are very inelastic, have a poor blood supply, and are difficult to repair when damaged. All stretches, therefore, should be felt *in the belly (centre) of the muscle* that is being stretched, rather than in the tendons.

Various researchers have observed that a muscle's responsiveness to stretch improves with increased temperature. It is advisable, therefore, to be warm before stretching and to maintain that warmth throughout the stretching session. Research suggests a temperature range of 103 – 114°F (40– 45°C) as optimal for maximum effect. In practical terms, this probably translates into feeling a 'glow' at the lower end of the temperature range (a useful guideline for warm-up stretches), and a feeling of 'gentle sweating' towards the upper range. When warm muscles are slowly stretched, the collagenous connective tissue, which is the most important limiting factor, seems to be affected most. Also, when warm collagenous connective tissue is stretched regularly, and for lengthy periods of time, there appears to be a relatively permanent change in its length, unlike muscle, which will always return to its resting length.

The other important factor in long-hold static stretching is time. How long is long? Although research findings vary, there is a degree of concensus towards 30–60 seconds. Individuals should progress in time and increase the length of the hold so gradually that discomfort is not felt, muscle spasms are avoided, and joints are not forced. Holding stretches for longer than a minute is also permissible when time allows. I advise people to stretch while watching TV or reading, and as part of relaxation. Long-hold stretching is very therapeutic, safe and effective. Music can often help create a good atmosphere for long-hold stretching, and is currently used by many athletes and exercise enthusiasts.

PARTNER STRETCHING

The aim of partner stretching is to introduce an element of teamwork into the process, which is both socially stimulating and effective in terms of increasing ROM. Partner stretches should be passive in nature; that is, the person being stretched should be completely relaxed, while the *stretcher* is the facilitator or helper – the one who does all the work.

It is important from the outset that the partners show care and consideration for each other, because sudden or vigorous movements can cause injury. In an environment of co-operation and trust, however, the benefits of partner stretching will be felt very effectively.

It is generally accepted that an individual's active range of movement is usually less than the passive range. While standing on one leg, flex the opposite knee and raise the heel into the bottom. When you hold this position you are stretching the quadriceps because of the contraction in the hamstrings (active stretch). Now take hold of the ankle, raise it slightly, and you will feel a greater stretch in the quadriceps because you are not relying on the strength of the hamstrings (passive stretch).

In partner stretching, the partner creates the passive stretch. This can be referred to, then, as *partner passive* stretching because it is the *stretcher* (not the performer) who promotes the increased range of movement. Once the performer is in the end position, the stretch is held for 30–60 seconds before the stretch is released. Stretches should be repeated up to four times per body part for optimum benefit.

Good communication is an important part of partner stretching so that the stretcher can receive feedback from the performer about how the stretch is progressing. In the event of any discomfort, the stretcher can ease off on the pressure, and if the position is being performed with ease, the stretch can be taken further.

PNF STRETCHES

PNF (see page 26) stretches are usually performed with a partner, but some of the personal stretches in the sections to follow can be converted into PNF stretches by following the principles that will be explained in that section.

Partner PNF stretches have two basic forms, but some specialists in massage therapy and physiotherapy use variations to promote specific results. The athlete can safely use the following techniques in the knowledge that they have been regarded by some researchers as the most advanced and effective techniques available for a healthy athlete with no injuries. Injured individuals, or those with medical problems, should always consult a physician before proceeding.

The two forms of PNF that are most useful to the athlete are the contract-relax method (CR) and the CRAC method.

Contract-Relax Method (CR Method)

When a muscle that is about to be stretched is contracted using an isometric (static) contraction, the GTO mechanism (*see* page 25) is engaged, resulting in greater relaxation of the muscle spindles and hence less resistance to stretching. This allows the muscle to stretch further than it would normally and thus permits a greater ROM in the joint. For this reason it is vital that the utmost care is taken by participants in the execution of the stretch, so that uncontrolled overstretching is avoided.

The procedure for the CR method is illustrated in fig 14a, but all the partner stretches in the relevant section can be converted into PNF stretches by following the contract-relax principles. In all cases the muscle that is about to be stretched is isometrically contracted against the resistance provided by the partner. This contraction should be held for 6 seconds, which is plenty of time to allow the golgi-tendon organs to react, but not long enough to have an adverse effect on blood pressure (long isometric contractions tend to increase blood pressure and thus are not recommended). Also, as a general principle, holding the breath is not advisable, because this causes an increase in intra-abdominal pressure; this can be useful in some weight-training movements when employed for short periods of time, but when sustained it is likely to increase pressure on the internal organs. Rhythmical breathing, therefore, should be encouraged at all times.

Once in the final stretch position, the stretch can be held for 30–60 seconds. It is possible, at this stage, to repeat the contract-relax procedure if a good response was not achieved the first time. A good response is characterized by the muscle completely yielding, offering no resistance to the movement being performed. The limb moves with much greater ease, and a much greater ROM is achieved. If this occurs on the first contract-relax procedure, then the end stretch position can be held for 30 – 60 seconds without repeating another isometric contraction.

In the partner stretch for the hamstrings shown in fig 14a, A lies supine with one hip flexed, and the knee of that leg comfortably straight. B kneels in front of A's straight leg, resting the calf of that leg on the shoulder. B now eases A's leg closer to A's chest until a mild stretch in A's hamstrings is felt. A now

pushes firmly against B's shoulder, but no movement should take place. This is an isometric contraction of the hamstrings, which is held for 6 seconds. A now stops pushing and after a brief (1 second) pause, B is able to ease A's leg closer to A's chest.

The CRAC Technique (Contraction, Relaxation, Agonist, Contraction)

To illustrate the CRAC technique, the example given in fig 14a can be used again. The contraction-relaxation phase is the same in CRAC as in the CR method. However, after the isometric contraction of A's hamstrings, A now moves the same leg towards her chest. The difference between CRAC and the CR method, then, is that A is active in the

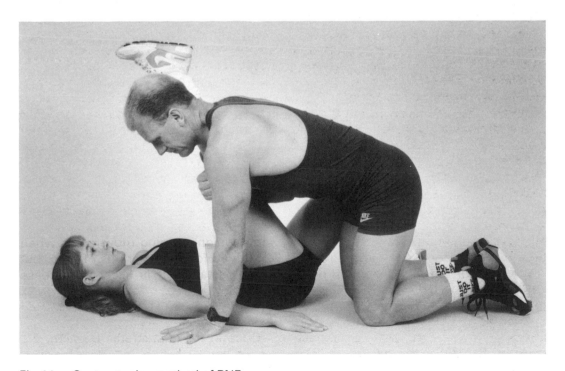

Fig 14a   Contract-relax method of PNF.

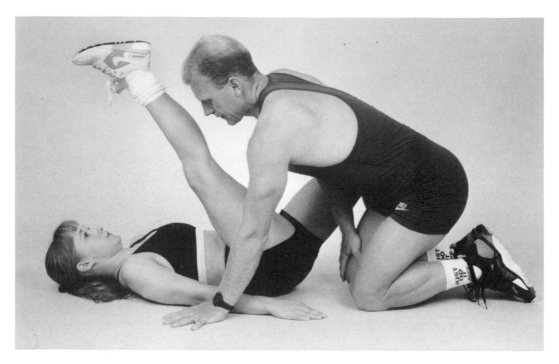

Fig 14b   CRAC PNF. The performer pulls her leg towards her face without assistance.

final part of the manoeuvre, that is, in producing the stretch (fig 14b). To move the leg to the chest, A contracts the hip flexor muscles and pulls the leg towards the chest – agonist contraction.

This method has the benefit of increasing the suppleness of the hamstrings (helped by the GTO response) by causing greater relaxation, and increasing the strength of the hip flexors. In addition, the active contraction of the hip flexors promotes reciprocal inhibition, discussed earlier. Remember, when one muscle (the agonist) contracts, its opposite (the antagonist) relaxes.

Once again, the partner stretches in the partner stretching section can be converted to CRAC stretches by following these principles.

4
Stretches to Avoid

Some stretches, as well as some *types* of stretching, are safer than others. Static stretching is now considered to be safer than dynamic stretching, for example, for the reasons explained earlier; however, it should be recognized that with any exercise there will always be a potential risk, which must be offset against the potential gain. Similarly, what is a safe stretch for one person may be unsafe for another owing to that individual's particular set of circumstances.

It is important that athletes carefully consider which stretches are most relevant to them, so that they obtain the maximum benefit and the minimum risk. The section on sport specific stretches will enable the performer to do this, but in the meantime it is worth considering some of the stretches that have received most criticism because of the stress they place on the body's structures, which could lead to injury.

It is strongly recommended that these stretches be eliminated from a performer's regime, and the reasons for exclusion are indicated alongside each particular stretch.

TOE-TOUCH STRETCH FOR THE HAMSTRINGS (Fig 15)
This stretch places the spine in a position of tremendous strain unless the hands can reach the floor and give

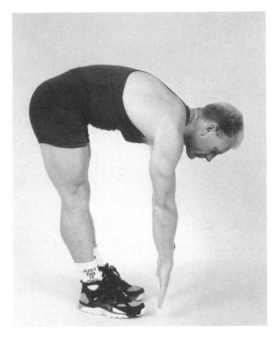

Fig 15   Toe-touch stretch.

support. The effectiveness of the stretch is also under question given that relaxation of the hamstrings is difficult because of the standing posture. Research into lower-back pain has indicated that the forward flexed position of the trunk places a severe load on the lumbar vertebrae, and that, as the trunk is lowered to a right-angle position, the muscular support is very limited, adding to the work that the ligaments must perform.

39

This posture is made worse if repeated bouncing actions are used to try to force a lower position of the hands. Not only does this increase the strain on the spine, but it also stimulates the myotatic reflex mechanism in the hamstring muscles. For safer alternatives to this position, refer to the short- and long-hold stretches for the hamstrings.

INNER THIGH AND HAMSTRING STRETCH
(Fig 16)
Again the spine is placed in an anatomically weak position so that the forces on it are great. In this stretch, however, with the arms outstretched, the lever is much longer than the example in fig 15, and therefore even more strain is created than in the toe-touch stretch. For safe alternatives to this stretch *see* figs 31 and 37 in the 'Short-Hold Stretches' section.

WINDMILL STRETCH TO MOBILIZE THE LOWER BACK AND STRETCH THE HAMSTRINGS
(Fig 17)
This exercise has been popular for some time but it is important to note that it places the spine in a position of great strain. While in this position the spine is rotated; unfortunately, because capacity for rotation in the lumbar (lower) spine is severely limited, the ligaments that hold the vertebrae together receive a strong rotational force. Rotation is a movement

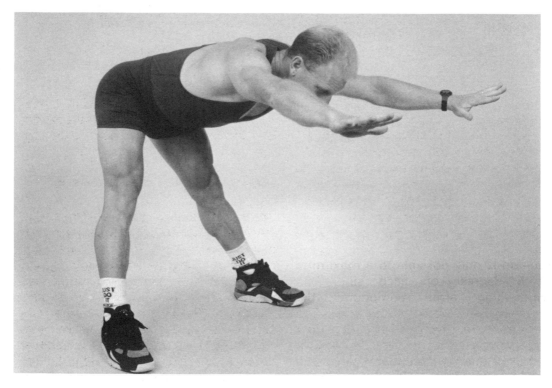

Fig 16   Inner thighs and hamstrings.

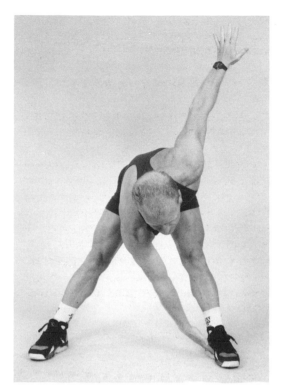

Fig 17   Windmill stretch.

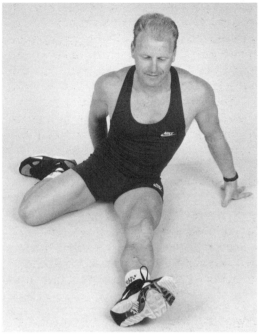

Fig 18   Hurdler's stretch.

the spinal column as a unit can perform, but different sections of the spine are only able to produce varying degrees of rotation. For example, rotation is most free in the cervical region; followed by the thoracic region. However, because of the interlocking of the articular surfaces (joint surfaces) in the lumbar region, rotation is only possible to a maximum of 5 degrees on each side. The windmilling arms compound the problem by adding momentum. The vertebrae are easily taken past their limited movement potential at speed, so it is clear that the potential for injury in this exercise is great. For safe ways to stretch the spine *see* figs 44 and 45 in the section on 'Long-Hold Stretching' and figs 98, 101 and 102 in the section on stretches for 'Running and Jumping Activities' in Chapter 6 (page 88).

HURDLER'S STRETCH FOR THE HIP REGION
(Fig 18)
This stretch places great strain on the knee of the bent leg, and while it may be appropriate for hurdlers, it can be avoided by using the stretches in figs 42 and 46 in the 'Long-Hold Stretches' section. The important question to ask yourself is, 'Why am I performing this stretch?' If the answer is to stretch the hamstrings, there is no reason to involve the knee of the opposite leg. If the answer is to replicate the action of the hurdling movement (because you are a

41

hurdler), there is probably more justification for using this stretch.

Recently, however, the value of this stretch to hurdlers has also been questioned, as it has been pointed out that a hurdler in flight does not have to cope with pressure on the bent knee from below. It is the hip abduction movement that needs to be free so that the trailing leg can clear the hurdle. The muscles that oppose abduction are, of course, the adductors, and they can be safely stretched without rotating the knee. It is the rotation of the bent knee in the hurdler's stretch that gives most concern because of the strain it places on the medial ligaments. This will not occur in free flight, owing to a lack of pressure from below. It therefore makes sense for a hurdler to concentrate on hamstring and inner thigh suppleness so that both movements are free when applied to the hurdling action.

THE PLOUGH FOR THE BACK, NECK AND HAMSTRINGS
(Fig 19)
This stretch places the cervical vertebrae of the neck in extreme hyperflexion, a position thought to be harmful because of the strain put on them. For alternatives, *see* figs 44 and 47 in the 'Long-Hold Stretches' section. Compression on the cervical vertebrae is particularly worrying as they are very small and easily damaged. Similarly, the position produces spinal and hip flexion, which, in the inverted position, can result in an uncomfortable squashing of the mid-section. This tends to cause a feeling of nausea.

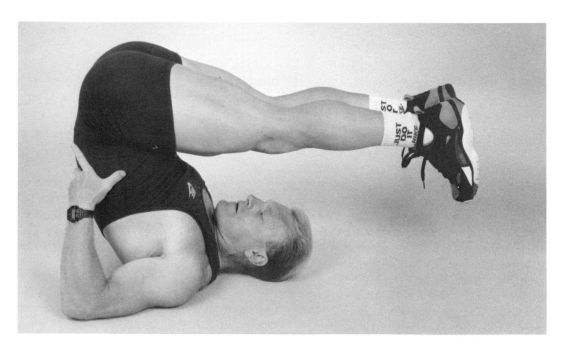

Fig 19   The plough.

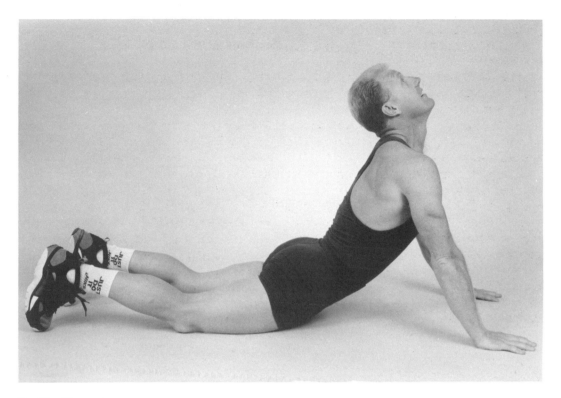

Fig 20   The cobra.

THE COBRA FOR THE ANTERIOR SPINE AND THE ABDOMINAL MUSCLES

(Fig 20)

This is a very severe stretch which impinges on the posterior aspect of the lumbar intervertebral discs and stretches the anterior portion. Severe strain is also placed on the neck, which is placed in hyperextension. For a safe alternative to this stretch see fig 51 in the section on 'Long-Hold Stretches'. In addition, it is worth noting that over-stretching the abdominals is not a desirable objective, since it is this practice in élite gymnasts that actually contributes to hyper-lordosis (abnormal curvature) in the spine, and consequently precipitates lower back pain, both while competing and in later life.

Extreme hyperextension of the spine is harmful; smaller ranges of movement can be tolerated more safely. The abdominal musculature can benefit from a small amount of stretching, but not the over-stretching that the cobra position creates, because one of the functions of the abdominals is to support the spine and help with good posture.

Having been shown some of the most severely criticized movements that are often seen in the preparation for sport, it is worthwhile for every athlete to look at their own practice to see whether the

43

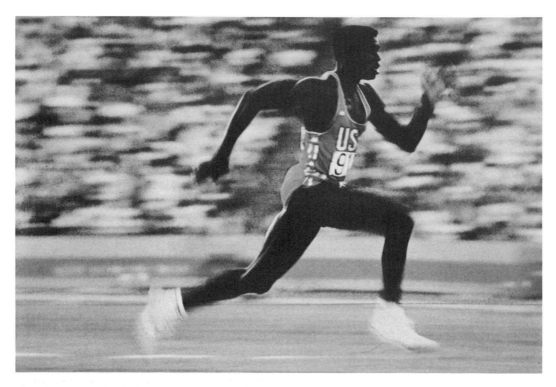

Exerting force through a greater range of movement can enhance performance, as in sprinting.

movements, exercises and postures they use are actually creating a harmful environment for the body rather than promoting a harmonious one. The arguments for and against an exercise being used will always involve a cost and benefit analysis. If the potential cost outweighs the potential benefit then the exercise should be rejected and an alternative found. There will always be safer alternatives and if they are equally effective they deserve serious consideration.

5

The Stretches

WARM-UP STRETCHING

Stretching should be an integral part of all warm-ups, but should not be performed while the body is cold. Short stretches lasting 8 – 10 seconds can be usefully performed after a period of 5 – 8 minutes of gentle rhythmical movements such as stepping, jogging, or skipping. This will provide a general warming of the body, which should then be followed by specific mobilization, that is, small movements in specific joints that are confined to the inner and middle ranges of that joint. These movements can include shoulder rolling, arm and knee bending, repeated hip flexion and extension, pelvic rotations and ankle movements.

By now the body will be ready to receive the benefit from short stretches which are designed primarily to facilitate greater relaxation in the muscle, and to achieve some gentle stretching of the structures to prepare them better for the task in hand. Stretching muscles in preparation for more vigorous activity will literally 'show the muscles the way' with regard to the movements they will be required to make later in the training session or performance. Muscle spindles will be better prepared and muscles and tendons will have achieved slightly greater elongation, which will also have

contributed to increasing the warmth of the tissues.

Following the stretching, a specific warm-up for the activity being undertaken should be included. This might be dribbling and shooting in basketball, stick-work in hockey, or easy hitting in tennis or squash. The aim of this part of the warm-up is specifically to practise the movement patterns in the sport or activity being prepared for. In a similar way, warm-up for a weight-training session would include the use of light weights at this stage. This kind of specific preparation has been referred to as preparing the neurological pathways, involving proprioception, innervation and co-ordination.

The performer should now be ready to begin the specific activity feeling well prepared and not at all fatigued. The total time of a warm-up varies from one activity to another depending on the severity of the effort, or, in the case of gymnastics, for example, on the complexity of the exercises. In the latter example, much more stretching would be performed than, for example, in the preparation for a bowls match. It is important to recognize, therefore, that fig 21 is only a guide, and individual activities may have their own modifications.

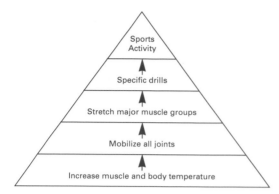

Fig 21   Stretching as part of a sport specific warm-up.

The following stretches are suitable for all sports participants. Most athletes will require a short-hold stretch of between 8 and 10 seconds per stretch. However, with sports such as gymnastics or swimming that demand high levels of flexibility, these same stretches can be progressed, repeated, and held for longer (30–60 seconds).

Short-Hold Stretches

The actual muscles are illustrated the first time they are mentioned in the text.

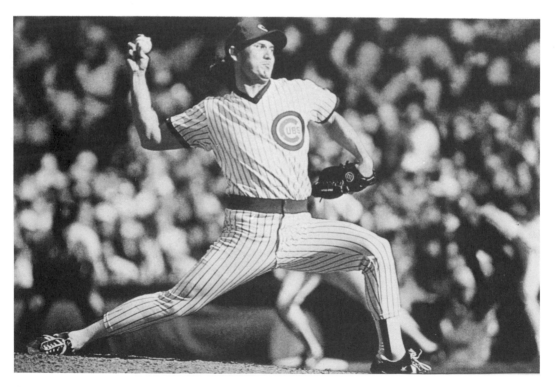

Good flexibility enhances throwing technique and may reduce the risk of injury.

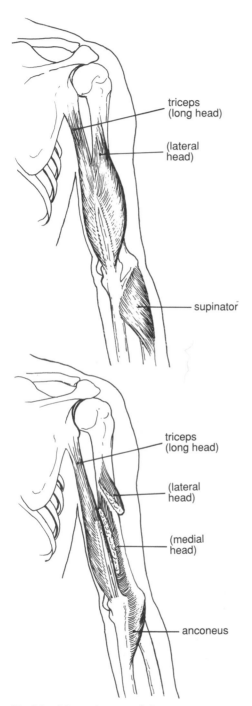

triceps
(long head)

(lateral
head)

supinator

triceps
(long head)

(lateral
head)

(medial
head)

anconeus

Fig 22 Musculature of the upper arm.

UPPER ARM STRETCH FOR THE TRICEPS
(Fig 23)
Take the arm above the head, bend the elbow, and gently pull the elbow down and back with the other hand. Pay attention to your posture; bend the knees, fix the pelvis, and do not arch the back. Repeat on the other side. This is a key stretch in elbow and shoulder flexibility, especially when it is realized that the long head of the triceps originates on the scapula. Tight triceps would be a major limitation in throwing events, gymnastics and swimming.

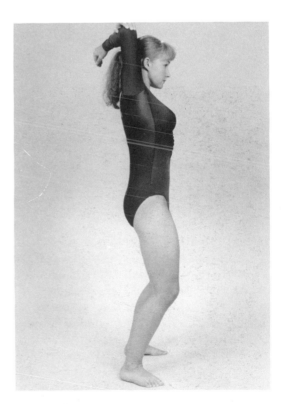

Fig 23 Upper arms.

47

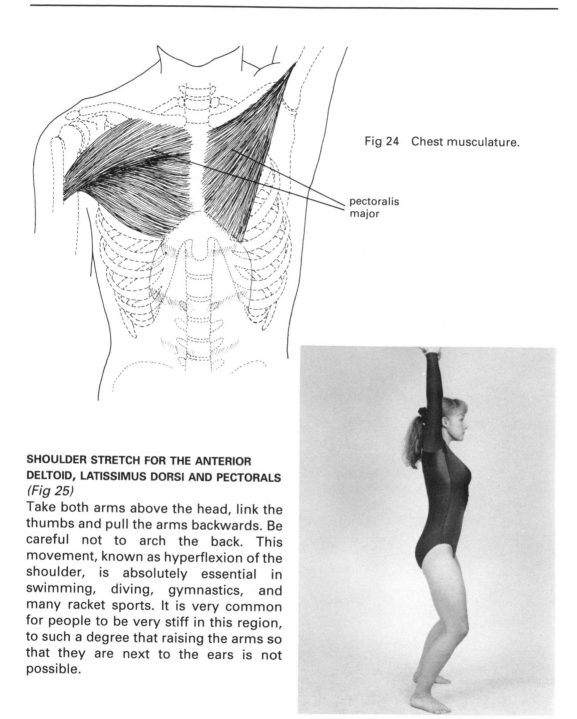

Fig 24   Chest musculature.

pectoralis
major

**SHOULDER STRETCH FOR THE ANTERIOR
DELTOID, LATISSIMUS DORSI AND PECTORALS
(Fig 25)**
Take both arms above the head, link the
thumbs and pull the arms backwards. Be
careful not to arch the back. This
movement, known as hyperflexion of the
shoulder, is absolutely essential in
swimming, diving, gymnastics, and
many racket sports. It is very common
for people to be very stiff in this region,
to such a degree that raising the arms so
that they are next to the ears is not
possible.

Fig 25   Shoulders.

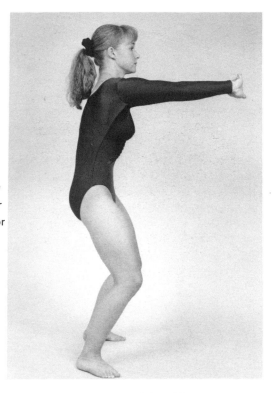

Fig 27 Upper back and shoulders.

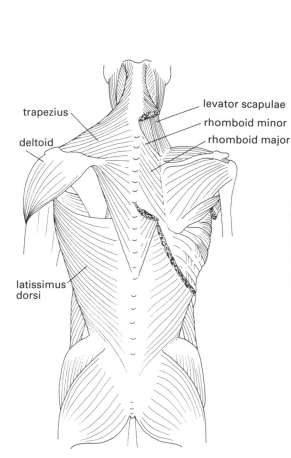

Fig 26 Back musculature.

UPPER BACK AND SHOULDER STRETCH
(Fig 27)
This stretches the rhomboids, trapezius 3 (between the scapulae) and posterior deltoid. Link the hands, push the arms in front of the chest. Pull the abdomen in, bend the knees and localize the stretch between the shoulder blades. The shoulder-blade area is a collecting point for tension, and this stretch in particular can help to relieve this. It also acts as a major postural stretch.

49

CHEST STRETCH FOR THE PECTORALIS MAJOR
(Fig 28)
Take the hands behind the back, link the hands and pull the arms back. Bend the knees and be sure not to lean forwards. Tight chest muscles may contribute to a round-shouldered posture and so it is important that the pectorals are stretched regularly. However, it is important to note that the muscle fibres of the pectoralis major actually run in three different directions, and because of this a number of different stretches can be used. This muscle was also stretched in fig 25, and in that stretch the majority of the sternal fibres were stretched.

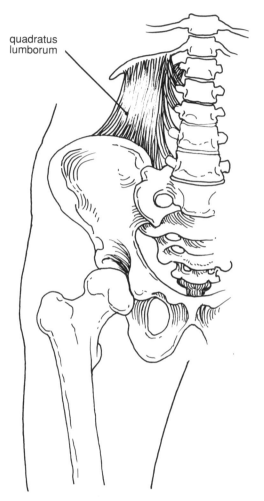

Fig 29   The quadratus lumborum.

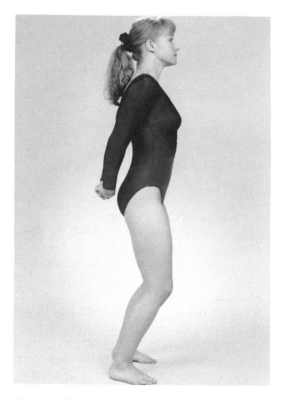

Fig 28   Chest.

SIDE STRETCH FOR THE QUADRATUS LUMBORUM, LATISSIMUS DORSI AND INTERCOSTALS
(Fig 30)
Bend the knees, fix the pelvis by pulling in the abdomen and place one hand on the hip. This hand is very important because it supports the body-weight.

50

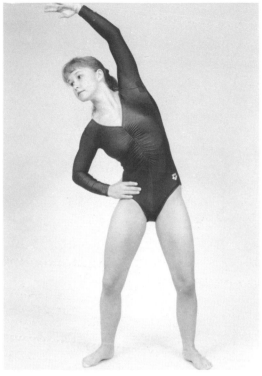

Fig 30   Sides.

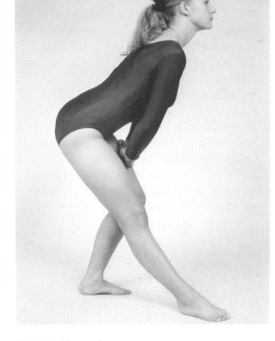

Fig 31   Upper legs.

With the weight on the hand on the hip, reach up with the other hand, and then reach over until a stretch is felt down the side. Repeat on the other side. If the body-weight is not supported in this stretch, the target muscles are not, in fact, stretched but eccentrically contracted. This means they are having to exert a lowering force to overcome the effects of gravity. Not only is this very hard work but it also puts strain on the lumbar spine and is therefore not recommended.

UPPER LEG STRETCH
(Fig 31)
This stretches the hamstrings – semi-membranosus, semitendinosus and biceps femoris. Take a step forwards with one leg, then bend the back leg. Place both hands on this leg to support the weight and protect the spine. Now lean forwards until a stretch is felt above the knee on the back of the front leg. Repeat on the other side. It is most important not to put the weight on the straight leg as this is likely to hyperextend the knee. Also, it is important to stretch one leg at a time only, so that the spine is protected and an effective stretch is achieved in the target muscle.

51

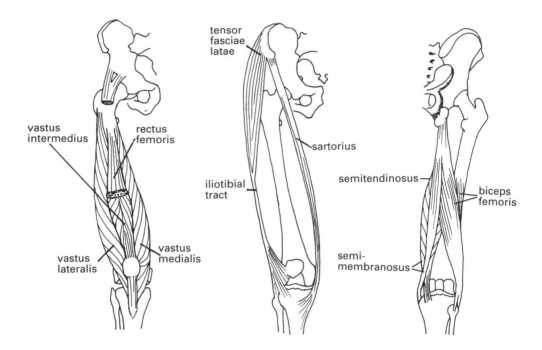

Fig 32   Thigh musculature.

THIGH STRETCH
(Fig 33)
This stretches the quadriceps-vastus medialis, vastus lateralis, vastus inter-medius and rectus femoris. Balance carefully on one leg. Use a wall for support if this is difficult. Bring the heel into the bottom, but keep the knees together (twisting the knee can injure it). Hold the ankle and push the hip forward. Take care not to pull the foot up to the bottom as this can over-stress the front of the knee. The main trauma is to the patella tendon and to the anterior cruciate ligaments, which are stretched when a deep knee flexion is attempted. This extreme position can be avoided by following the instructions above. Repeat on the other side.

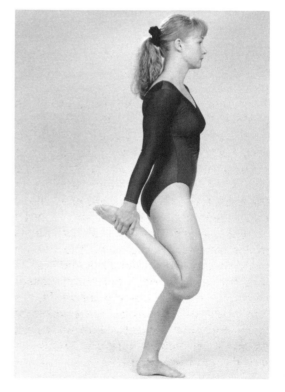

Fig 33   Thighs.

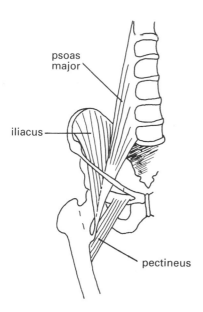

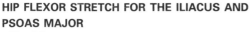

Fig 34   Deep hip flexor muscles.

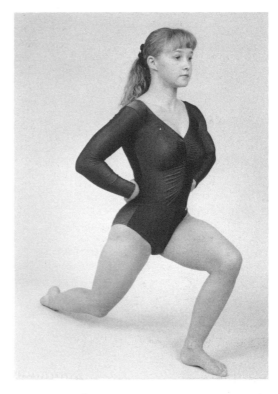

Fig 35   Hip flexors.

HIP FLEXOR STRETCH FOR THE ILIACUS AND PSOAS MAJOR
(Fig 35)
Take a step forwards, but not so far as to achieve less than a right angle at the front knee. Then lower the pelvis towards the floor, bending the rear knee at the same time. Feel the stretch on the front of the hip but take care not to arch the back. Repeat on the other side. Many people lean forwards in this stretch but it is worth remembering that the psoas major muscle originates on the twelfth thoracic and lumbar vertebra and inserts into the top of the inner thigh (lesser trochanter); so by leaning forwards, the two ends of this muscle are brought closer together rather than further apart, as in a stretch. Therefore, keep an upright posture as shown.

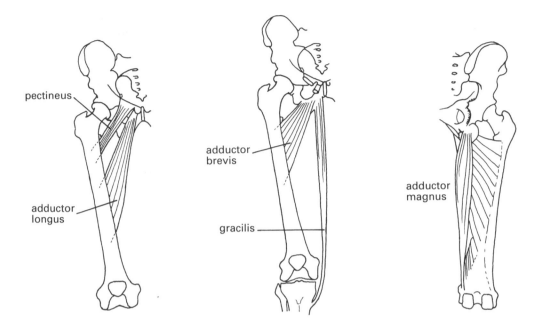

Fig 36   Adductor muscles of the thigh.

INNER THIGH STRETCH FOR THE ADDUCTORS, PECTINEUS AND GRACILIS
(Fig 37)
Step to the side with one leg and bend that knee so that the knee is over the big toe and not twisted. The other leg is kept straight and a stretch is felt in the inner thigh. Be careful not to bend forwards, or to allow the foot of the straight leg to turn inwards as this will strain the knee at the medial ligaments. Repeat on the other side.

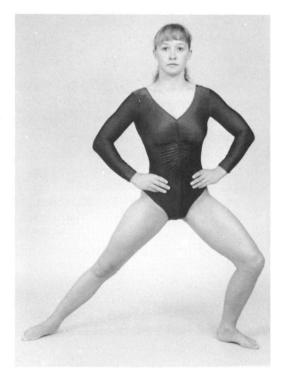

Fig 37   Inner thighs.

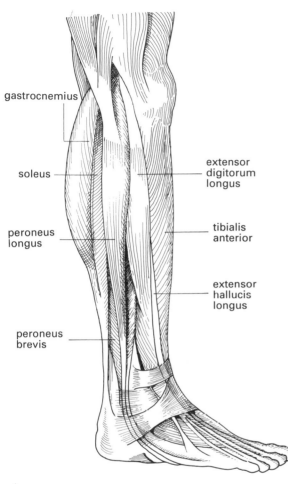

gastrocnemius

soleus

peroneus
longus

peroneus
brevis

extensor
digitorum
longus

tibialis
anterior

extensor
hallucis
longus

Fig 38   Muscles of the lower leg.

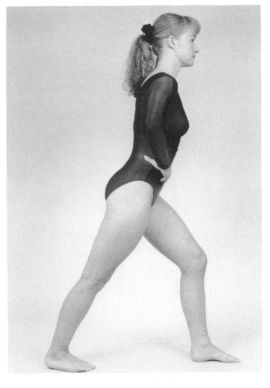

Fig 39   Calves.

CALF STRETCH FOR THE GASTROCNEMIUS
(Fig 39)

Take a small step forwards and bend the front knee. Push the rear heel into the floor making sure the foot points forwards. A stretch is felt at the back of the lower leg. Repeat on the other side. It is important that the knee of the rear leg is kept straight so that the gastrocnemius, which also crosses the knee, is fully stretched.

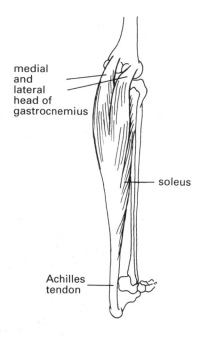

medial
and
lateral
head of
gastrocnemius

soleus

Achilles
tendon

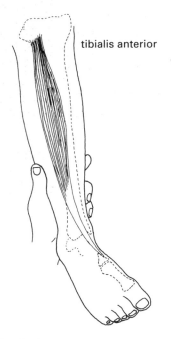

tibialis anterior

Fig 40   Calf muscles.

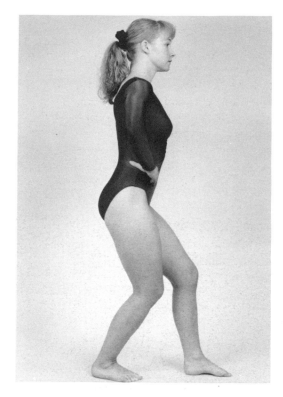

Fig 41   Lower calves.

LOWER-CALF STRETCH
(Fig 41)
This stretches the soleus, tibialis posterior, flexor digitorum longus and flexor hallucis longus (situated beneath the gastrocnemius). From the calf stretch in fig 39, bend the rear knee so that the patella moves towards the floor. This will move the stretch from the calf to the lower calf. Repeat on the other side. This is an especially important stretch for runners, games players and skiers. Runners become very tight in this region owing to the repeated contractions of these muscles when pounding the streets, and skiers need to get well forwards in their boots to achieve a good skiing posture.

Long-Hold Stretches

Hold these stretches for a minimum of 30–60 seconds, increasing the time as you feel more comfortable. It is important to concentrate on lengthening the muscle, but no pain should be felt. If the muscle appears to relax a little during the stretch, ease a little further into the stretch so that the intensity is maintained. These stretches can be repeated as often as you like and can be used on a daily basis provided you are warm.

These stretches focus on the lower body and are supported so that comfort and relaxation are achieved. Therefore, always perform these stretches on a mat or carpet. Some of the stretches can be converted to PNF stretches, and instructions for doing so are given where appropriate.

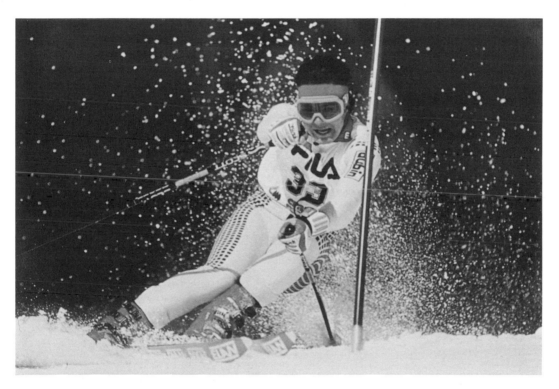

The all-round flexibility demands of skiing are illustrated in the slalom where angulation is a vital component.

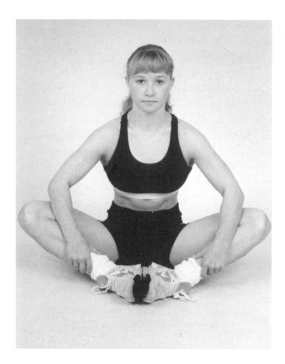

Fig 42   Inner thighs.

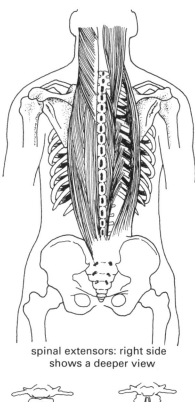

spinal extensors: right side
shows a deeper view

INNER THIGH STRETCH
(Fig 42)
This stretches the adductors – magnus
longus and brevis, pectineus and gracilis.
Sit tall with the soles of the feet together.
Rest the hands on the ankles but do not
pull on the feet. Press the knees
outwards with the elbows. To make this
a PNF stretch, squeeze the knees against
the elbows for 6 seconds, release, then
push the knees further apart. The groin
is a notoriously tight area in games
players and a common site for injury.
Regular stretching of this area is
therefore essential for improved
performance and perhaps for injury
prevention.

deep posterior muscles
of the spine

Fig 43   Muscles of the spine.

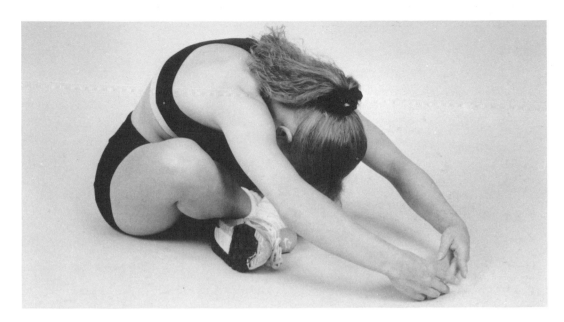

Fig 44   Lower back.

LOWER BACK STRETCH FOR THE ERECTOR SPINAE
(Fig 44)
Individuals may also feel this stretch in the buttocks and the inner thighs. Sit with legs crossed and lean slowly forwards allowing the chin to fall on to the chest. Relax and enjoy this position. If the stretch is difficult, place the hands behind the back on the floor, and push gently forwards. Many muscles make up the erector spinae group and are shown in fig 43.

SIDE STRETCH FOR THE QUADRATUS LUMBORUM, LATISSIMUS DORSI AND INTERCOSTALS
(Fig 45)
Sit comfortably; crossed legs are not essential. Place one hand on the floor next to the hip, stretch tall with the other hand and reach over. The hand on the floor is necessary to support the weight and protect the spine. Repeat on the other side.

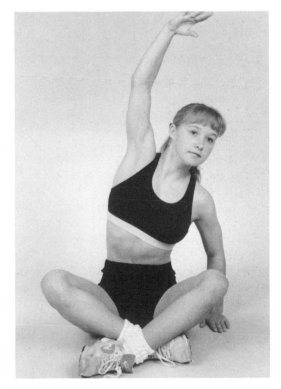

Fig 45   Sides.

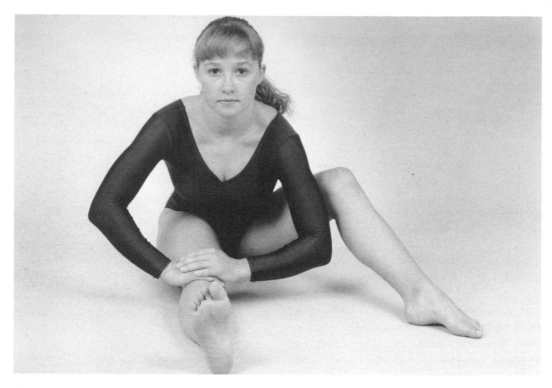

Fig 46   Hamstrings.

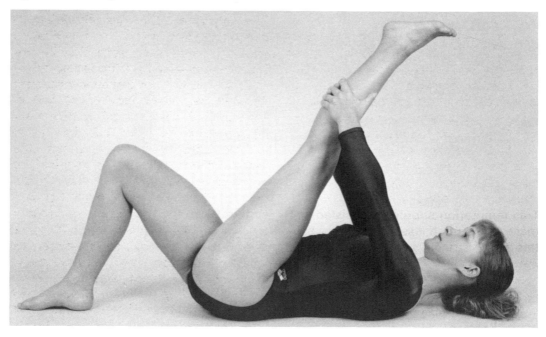

Fig 47   Hamstrings (variation).

HAMSTRING STRETCH FOR SEMIMEMBRANOSUS, SEMITENDINOSUS, AND BICEPS FEMORIS
(Fig 46)

Sit with one leg forwards, toe pointed to the ceiling. The other leg is out to the side where it is comfortable, and plays no part in the stretch. Lift tall from the hips and lean forwards, leading with the chin. There is no need to drop the head and flex the spine; you should feel the stretch at the back of the upper leg. Repeat on the other side. The position of the pelvis is very important in hamstring stretching. It should be tilted anteriorly (forwards) so that the upper part of the pelvis is forward and the lower part pushed down and back. This ensures that the two ends of the hamstring muscles are as far apart as possible, and hence fully stretched.

HAMSTRING STRETCH VARIATION
(Fig 47)

Lie with the back flat on the floor, bend one knee and place the foot of that leg close to the buttocks. Lift the other leg and hold the calf with both hands. If this is difficult, bend the knee slightly, or use a towel, a technique which is shown in fig 91 in Chapter 6. Ease the leg towards the face and feel a stretch above the knee at the back of the leg. Repeat on the other side. There is a tendency with this stretch to lift the bottom off the floor. This temptation should be resisted as it makes the stretch less effective. To make this a PNF stretch, push the calf against the hands for 6 seconds, release and ease the leg further towards the face. Be careful not to hold your breath, but breathe rhythmically throughout.

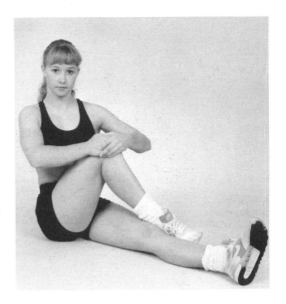

Fig 48   Outer hips.

OUTER HIP STRETCH
(Fig 48)

This stretches the hip abductors – gluteus medius, minimus, tensor fascia latae and the iliotibial band. Sit with one leg forwards and the other leg across it. Hold the outside of the knee and ease the bent leg across the chest and in towards it. A stretch is felt on the outer hip. Repeat on the other side. To convert this to a PNF stretch, simply push the bent leg away from the body against the immovable resistance of the hands. Push for 6 seconds, release and stretch further by taking the leg across and into the chest. The iliotibial band is not a muscle, but a fibrous band of connective tissue which runs down the outside of the thigh. It can become very tight with running and jumping activities and stretching it often gives a feeling of pleasant relief.

61

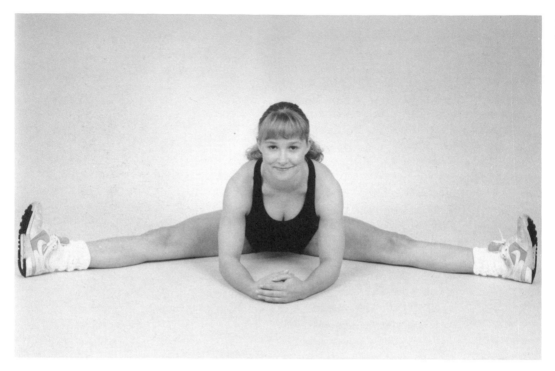

Fig 49   Advanced combination hip stretch.

ADVANCED COMBINATION HIP STRETCH
(Fig 49)

This stretches the hamstrings, adductors, gluteals and lower back. Sit with legs apart and toes turned upwards. Lean forwards slowly until a stretch is felt. Because this stretch affects a number of muscles, individuals will feel the stretch in different places. For many people this stretch may be too difficult and therefore should only be used if it feels comfortable. It will normally be an essential stretch in sports like gymnastics, skating and the martial arts.

FRONT SPINE AND ABDOMINAL STRETCH
(Fig 51)

Because the abdominals do not need a great deal of stretching, and because too much hyperextension (back arching) can be dangerous for the spine, only a small angle between the body and the floor is required in this stretch (30–45 degrees). Therefore, rest on the forearms, and push the sternum (breastbone) forwards, rather than looking up and straining the neck. It is interesting that in gymnastics, extreme hyperextension is thought to contribute to lower back pain for the gymnast in later life. We can learn from this information and ensure that we only stretch the structures that require stretching, and protect the ones that do not.

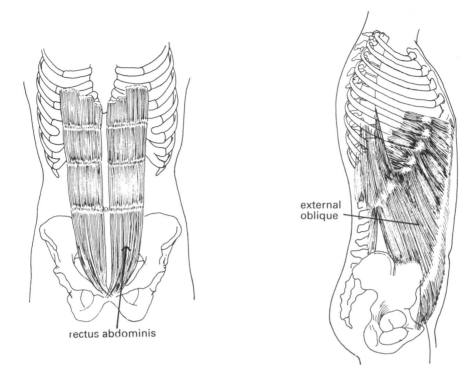

Fig 50   Muscles of the front of the trunk.

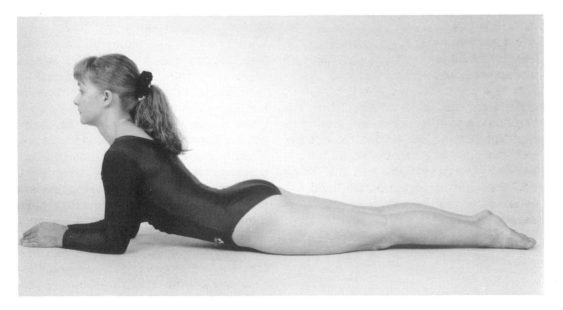

Fig 51   Front spine and abdominals.

63

PARTNER STRETCHES

The following stretches are performed with a partner and are excellent for developing flexibility in a relaxed, caring environment as part of a specific training session on flexibility, possibly performed in the home and aided by some appropriate music. The participants need to be very warm and ideally to have progressed through the short- and long-hold stretches already covered. Partner stretching is a natural development of these techniques.

In this section the person who is receiving the stretch (the performer) should be totally relaxed. The performer is completely passive in the movements, and the stretcher does all the work. It is essential, therefore, that all movements are performed very slowly and that good communication takes place between the individuals concerned. Conversions to PNF stretches are indicated as before.

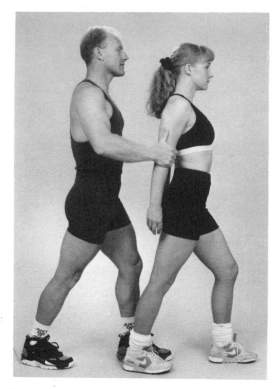

Fig 52   Chest and calves.

CHEST AND CALF STRETCH FOR THE PECTORALIS MAJOR, ANTERIOR DELTOID AND GASTROCNEMIUS
(Fig 52)
Stand one behind the other, one leg fowards, the other back so that both participants feel a calf stretch. The stretcher now holds the arms above the elbow of the person in front and eases the arms back to feel a stretch on the chest. It is important to hold the arms above the elbows so as not to strain them. To convert this to a PNF stretch, push the arms outwards against the resistance for 6 seconds before releasing and stretching further by bringing the elbows closer together. At the same time, push the ball of the rear foot firmly into the floor to contract the calf that is currently being stretched. After pushing for 6 seconds, release the pressure and further stretch will be created. Repeat the chest stretch and change legs.

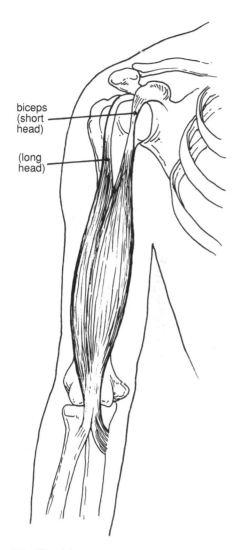

biceps
(short
head)

(long
head)

Fig 53 The biceps.

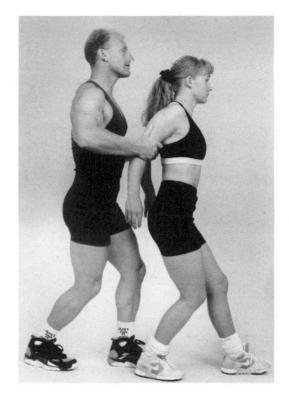

Fig 54 Upper chest and lower calves.

UPPER CHEST AND LOWER CALF STRETCH
(Fig 54)
This stretches the clavicular portion of the pectoralis major, the anterior deltoid and the short head of the biceps, as in fig 52, except that both individuals bend their rear legs so that the stretch is felt on the lower calf, and the elbow points are lifted upwards before they are brought backwards to feel the stretch on the upper chest. To convert to a PNF stretch the procedure is the same as in fig 52. Repeat the stretch and change legs. The biceps muscle is normally quite difficult to stretch, but because the short head originates on the coracoid process (point) of the scapula on the front of the shoulder, this position, which extends the shoulder, gives a useful stretch to the area. This is a common site of injury, particularly in swimmers and gymnasts because of over-stretching, so the musculature of this region has to be stretched with complete control to prevent injury.

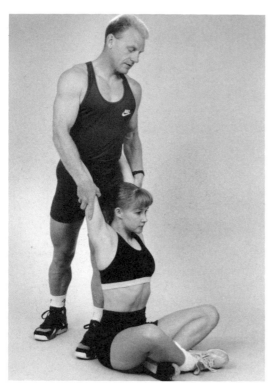

Fig 55   Shoulders.

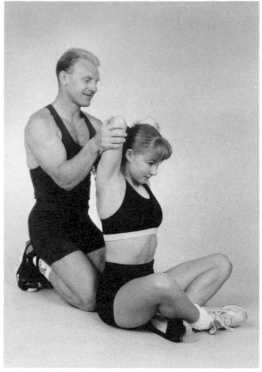

Fig 56   Under arms.

SHOULDER STRETCH FOR THE ANTERIOR DELTOID, LATISSIMUS DORSI AND PECTORALIS MAJOR
(Fig 55)
The stretcher stands side-on behind the performer so that the performer has a comfortable back rest. The arms are raised above the head and held above the elbows on the upper-arm bone (humerus). They are then eased backwards, taking care not to arch the back. To convert to a PNF stretch, the performer pushes forwards against the partner's resistance for 6 seconds before releasing and stretching further.

UNDER-ARM STRETCH FOR THE LATISSIMUS DORSI
(Fig 56)
While sitting comfortably, with a tall spine, the performer takes the arms above the head, bends the elbows, and places the palms of the hands on the nape of the neck. The elbows are now pointing upwards and the chin is on the chest. The stretcher now eases the elbow points together so a stretch is felt under the arms. To convert this to a PNF stretch, the performer pushes the elbows outwards against the stretcher's resistance for 6 seconds before releasing and stretching further. For an advanced version of this stretch, see fig 69 in the 'Stretching for Aquatic Activities' section in Chapter 6.

LOWER-BACK STRETCH FOR THE ERECTOR SPINAE
(Fig 57)

The performer sits with crossed legs and leans forwards. The stretcher places one hand on each scapula and pushes gently downwards, without body-weight. Participants should proceed with caution if a PNF version is to be attempted, and anyone with a back problem should not use the PNF alternative. To convert to a PNF stretch, the performer tries to sit up against the resistance. This is held for 6 seconds before release and the performer is eased further to the ground. It is important that both individuals stop pushing at the same time in order to avoid an action-reaction situation, which could result in injury.

INNER-THIGH STRETCH FOR THE ADDUCTORS, PECTINEUS AND GRACILIS
(Fig 58)

The performer sits with the soles of the feet together, knees apart. The stretcher kneels behind and places one hand on the inside of each knee before pushing gently downwards. To convert this to a PNF stretch, the performer squeezes the knee inwards against the stretcher's hands for 6 seconds before continuing the stretch. It is important to note that the performer will be much stronger than the stretcher in this position (arms versus legs), and so tension should be built together so that no movement is achieved in the contraction phase. Also, when the performer stops pushing, the stretcher must stop as well to avoid an action-reaction, which would produce a rapid stretch of the inner-thigh muscles, possibly causing injury.

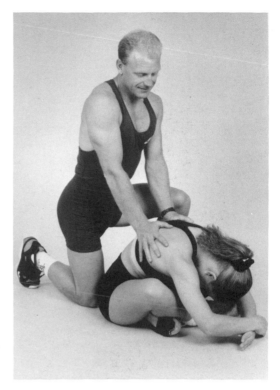

Fig 57   Lower back.

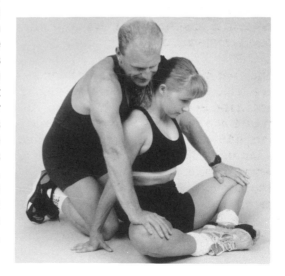

Fig 58   Inner thighs.

67

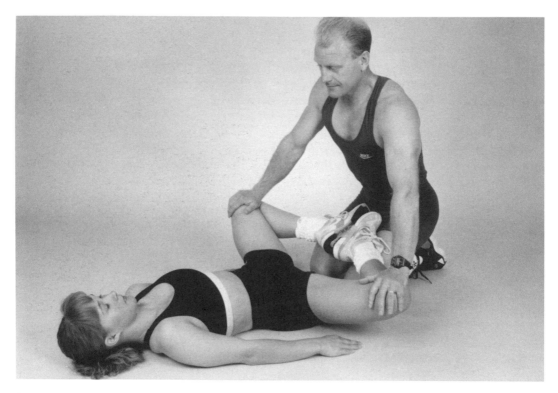

Fig 59   Inner thighs (advanced).

ADVANCED INNER-THIGH STRETCH FOR THE ADDUCTORS, PECTINEUS AND GRACILIS
(Fig 59)

As in fig 58, except the performer's feet are placed on the stretcher's thighs, while the performer is lying down. This position is excellent preparatory stretching for those wishing to progress towards a splits position, or for those who have particularly tight inner-thigh muscles. It is important that the performer's back is flat whilst lying down and that the thighs are in line with the pelvis, so that the stretch is localized. The next stage, one step closer to the splits position, is to perform the same stretch with the legs straight and the stretcher's hands placed just above the inside of the knees.

HAMSTRING STRETCH FOR SEMIMEMBRANOSUS, SEMITENDINOSUS AND BICEPS FEMORIS
(Fig 60)

The performer lies flat with one leg bent and the other straight. The straight leg is raised towards the chest. The stretcher now kneels in front of the straight leg and places a shoulder on the calf muscle. One of the stretcher's hands is placed on the floor for safety reasons and the other maintains a comfortably straight knee for the performer. The stretcher now moves slowly forwards

68

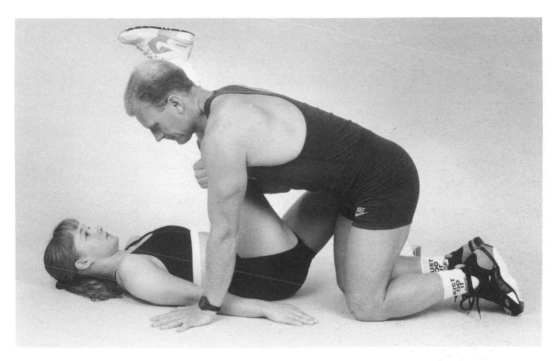

Fig 60 Hamstrings.

producing a stretch in the performer's hamstrings. For those wishing to advance towards the splits position in gymnastics or championship aerobics, for example, the bent leg can be straightened to achieve a specific stretch for splits.

To convert this to a PNF stretch, the performer pushes the calf against the stretcher's shoulder, thus contracting the hamstring muscles. After 6 seconds the push is released and the muscle is stretched further. With very flexible individuals it may be impractical for the stretcher to have the shoulder on the performer's calf muscle, because this may mean that the stretcher is literally lying on top of the performer. In this case, the stretcher's hand can be placed on the performer's calf. It will now be essential, however, that the limb is moved in a straight line and not allowed to wobble from side to side.

6
Sport Specific Stretches

The following stretches are arranged as specific stretches for groups of sports. It is intended that these stretches supplement the stretches already shown so that complete flexibility is developed, while at the same time catering for any specific needs of a particular sport. The sports groups are as follows: aquatics, which includes swimming, water polo and diving; racket/implement games, including squash, badminton, tennis, golf and cricket; team games, including soccer, hockey, netball, volleyball and rugby; and running/jumping sports.

Some sporting movements replicate positions that can be prepared for in training. A gradual and progressive development of these positions, provided they do not contra-indicate the body's natural potential for movement, should help to prepare the athlete better to be more effective in their movement performance, and may also help in the prevention of injury.

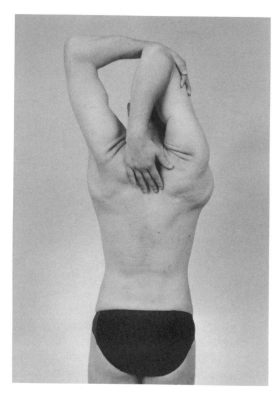

Fig 61   Triceps and latissimus dorsi.

STRETCHING FOR AQUATIC ACTIVITIES

BEHIND-THE-NECK STRETCH FOR THE TRICEPS AND LATISSIMUS DORSI
(Fig 61)
Because extreme flexibility is required, particularly in swimming, water polo and synchronized swimming, this stretch is very beneficial. Take the arm above the head with the elbow flexed. Pull the elbow back and across with the other hand, taking care not to arch the back in the process. Repeat on the other side. To convert to a PNF stretch, push the elbow into the hand. Hold this for 6 seconds, release, and continue the stretch.

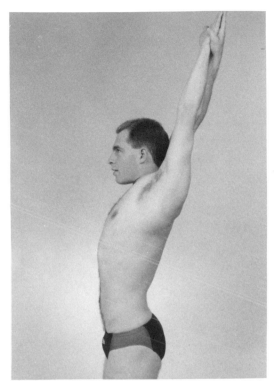

Fig 62   Shoulder hyperflexion.

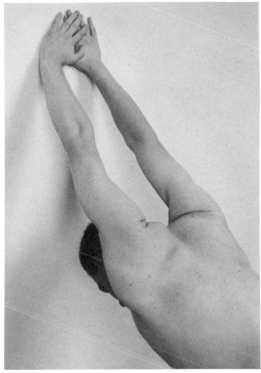

Fig 63   Hyperflexion against a wall.

SHOULDER HYPERFLEXION STRETCH FOR THE ANTERIOR DELTOID AND PECTORALS
(Fig 62)
Take the arms above the head, cross the hands, then press the arms backwards. This is an excellent stretch for simulating a streamline position, for example when pushing off the wall and gliding through the water.

HYPERFLEXION AGAINST A WALL, AS A DEVELOPMENT OF FIG. 62
(Fig 63)
Cross the hands and press the forehead towards the wall. To convert this into a PNF stretch, push against the wall for 6 seconds, release and press the forehead closer to the wall. Take care not to hyperextend the elbows. It is also worth noting that this stretch can be performed using a wall bar in a gym, or using the pool side while standing in the water.

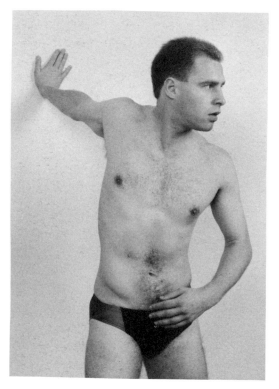

Fig 64   Chest.

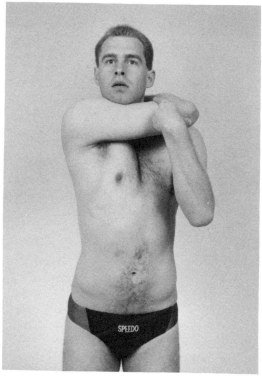

Fig 65   Backs of the shoulders.

CHEST STRETCH FOR THE PECTORALS AND THE ANTERIOR DELTOID
(Fig 64)
Place the hand flat against a wall and move the shoulder gently forwards. To convert to a PNF stretch, push against the wall for 6 seconds before releasing and pushing the shoulder further forwards. Repeat on the other side. Take care not to hyperextend the elbow.

BACK OF THE SHOULDER STRETCH FOR THE POSTERIOR DELTOID
(Fig 65)
Take the arm across the throat and hold it with the other arm. To convert to a PNF stretch, push back against the hand to contract the posterior deltoid, then release and continue the stretch. Repeat on the other side. Tight posterior deltoid muscles can be a major limiting factor to efficient swimming technique, and so a good deal of attention should be paid to this and the whole of the shoulder region.

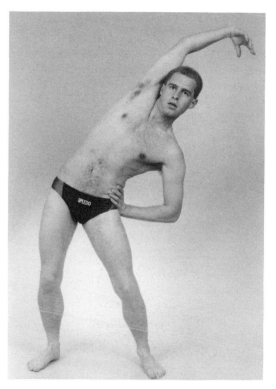

Fig 66   Sides.

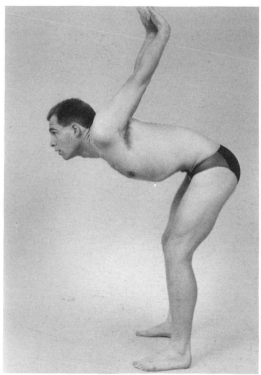

Fig 67   Chest and shoulders.

SIDE STRETCH FOR THE QUADRATUS LUMBORUM AND LATISSIMUS DORSI
(Fig 66)
Keeping the knees bent, take the arm above the head, and bend from the waist. The lower hand supports the weight. Repeat on the other side. The action of reaching to gain maximum potential in throwing or swimming, will be inhibited if the muscles of the side of the upper back (latissimus dorsi) and the side of the lower spine (quadratus lumborum) are not supple enough.

CHEST AND SHOULDER STRETCH FOR THE DELTOIDS, PECTORALS AND ROTATOR CUFF MUSCLES
(Fig 67)
The safe positioning of the spine here is of paramount importance. Bend the knees and push the pelvis down and back. Pull the abdominals in and hyperextend the shoulders as shown. If a comfortable position of the spine cannot be achieved, lie face down on a bench to perform this shoulder stretch.

73

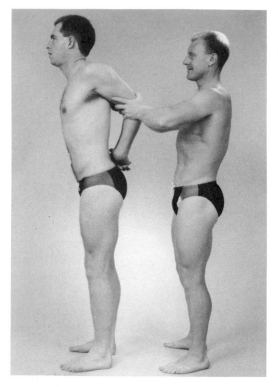

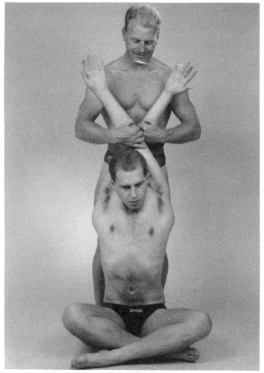

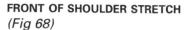
Fig 68   Front of the shoulders.

Fig 69   Shoulders.

FRONT OF SHOULDER STRETCH
(Fig 68)
This stretches the clavicular portion of the pectoralis major, the anterior deltoid and the short head of the biceps. The arms are taken back by a partner and then lifted upwards. The performer pushes outwards against the stretcher's hands for 6 seconds, and following the release of this contraction, the muscles are stretched further.

SHOULDER STRETCH FOR THE LATISSIMUS DORSI AND PECTORALS
(Fig 69)
The performer takes the arms above the head and crosses them. The stretcher holds the humerus of both arms so that the elbows are not strained, and eases the arms across one another. An easier version of this stretch is shown in fig 56 of the 'Partner Stretches' section in Chapter 5.

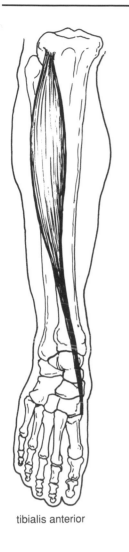

tibialis anterior

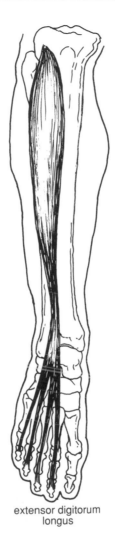

extensor digitorum
longus

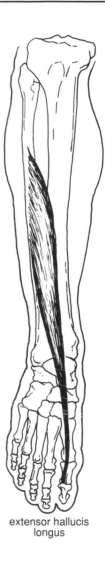

extensor hallucis
longus

Fig 70   Shin and toe musculature.

ANKLE STRETCH
(Fig 71)
This stretches the extensor digitorum longus (little toe extensors), tibialis anterior (shin muscle) and extensor hallucis longus (big toe extensor). While sitting, take one foot across the other, flex the ankle (which is then plantar flexed), and point (flex) the toes. Create further flexion by using the hand.

ANKLE STRETCH VARIATION
(Fig 72)
While sitting with the legs straight, point the toes and plantar flex the ankles. Push one foot down with the other. A PNF

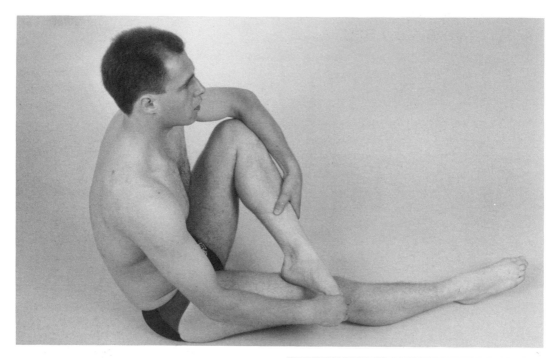

Fig 71   Ankles.

variation of this is to pull upwards against the top foot with the lower foot for 6 seconds before releasing and continuing the stretch.

Perhaps the most effective ankle stretch is to kneel on a cushion and sit on your heels. However, this can place a strain on the knees and so is not suitable for everyone. There is no point improving the flexibility in one joint at the cost of damaging another. As an alternative, try lying face downwards with the feet on a pillow that has been bent in half. Push the feet into the pillow with pointed toes.

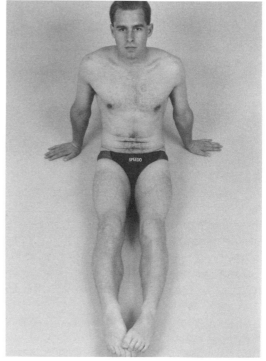

Fig 72   Ankles (variation).

STRETCHING FOR RACKET/IMPLEMENT SPORTS

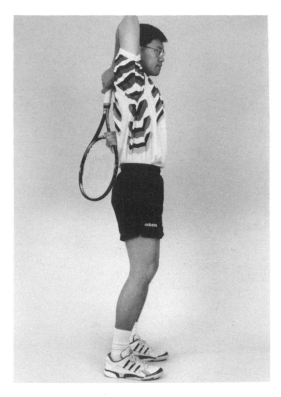

Fig 73   Triceps stretch with implement.

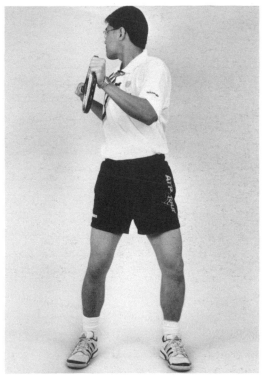

Fig 74   Oblique stretch.

TRICEPS STRETCH WITH IMPLEMENT
(Fig 73)
Keep the knees bent and be careful not to arch the back. Take one arm above the head, flex the elbow, and let the weight of the racket produce a gentle stretch. Pull down on the racket to increase the stretch. Repeat on the other side.

OBLIQUE STRETCH
(Fig 74)
Keep the knees and hips pointing forwards as the racket is held across the chest. Without swinging, rotate the spine and look over your shoulder. Return to face front before repeating on the other side. This is an essential stretch to be performed before any hitting techniques are used, but it *must* be performed with control.

77

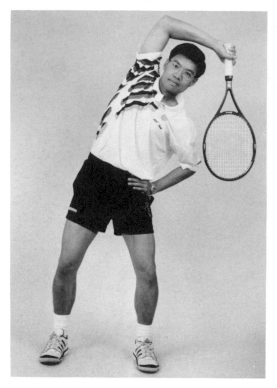

Fig 75   Quadratus lumborum.

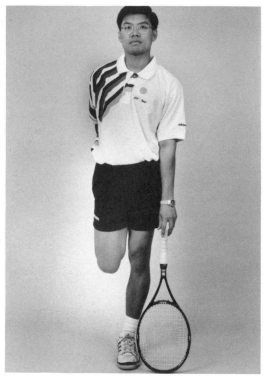

Fig 76   Quadriceps.

QUADRATUS LUMBORUM STRETCH
(Fig 75)
With the knees bent and the pelvis fixed in a neutral position, take the racket above the head, flex the elbow, and support the body with the other hand. The weight of the racket helps to increase the stretch. Repeat on the other side.

QUADRICEPS STRETCH
(Fig 76)
Use the implement for support, bend the supporting leg to aid balance, and raise the heel of the other leg towards the buttocks. Hold the ankle, but push the hip forwards, rather than pull the heel to the bottom. Repeat on the other side.

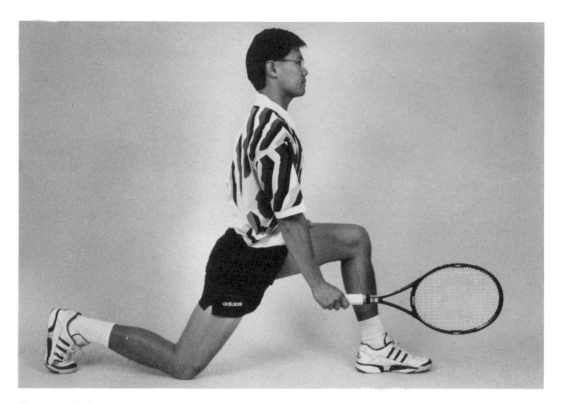

Fig 77   Hip flexors.

HIP FLEXOR STRETCH
(Fig 77)
All sports that use a lunge position could usefully employ this stretch. It is important, however, that the front knee shows a right angle, and that the pelvis moves downwards and not forwards as you ease into the stretch. Keep the trunk upright at all times. The main stretch is felt on the top of the thigh on the rear leg (hip flexors). Repeat on the other side.

79

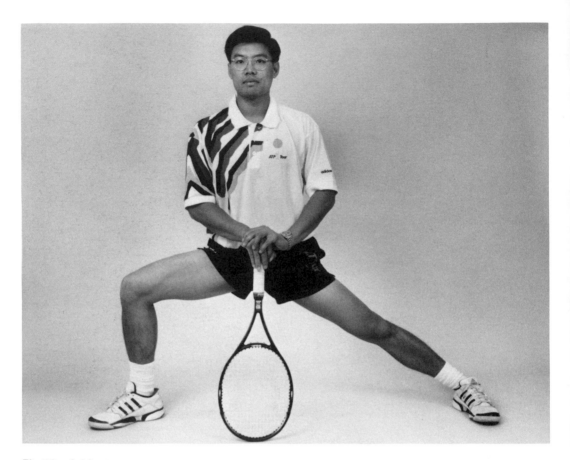

Fig 78   Adductors.

ADDUCTOR STRETCH
(Fig 78)
Using the racket for support, bend one knee to a right angle and take the other leg to the side, foot pointing to the front. The stretch is felt on the inner thigh of the straight leg. Repeat on the other side. Be careful not to let the foot of the straight leg roll inwards. Strained groin muscles are very common in implement sports, especially in tennis, squash, badminton and cricket. Regular stretching will help promote the well-being of this area.

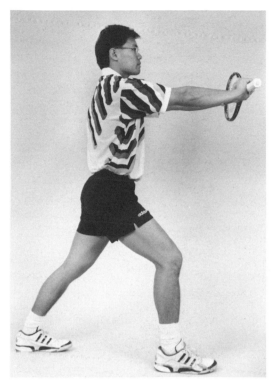

Fig 79   Gastrocnemius and rhomboids.

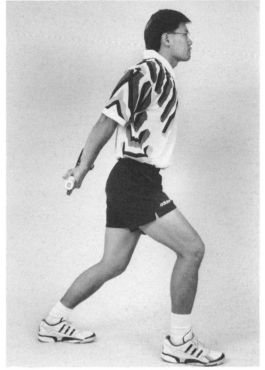

Fig 80   Pectorals and lower calves.

GASTROCNEMIUS AND RHOMBOID STRETCH
(Fig 79)

Take a step backwards and point the rear foot forwards. Bend the front knee so that you feel a stretch in the rear calf. At the same time, hold the racket in front of the chest, and push the arms away from the body to feel the stretch across the back of the shoulder blades. Repeat with the other leg back.

PECTORALS AND LOWER-CALF STRETCH
(Fig 80)

As in fig 79, except the rear knee is bent, and in this stretch the racket is held behind the back so that it can be lifted away from the body to produce a chest stretch.

81

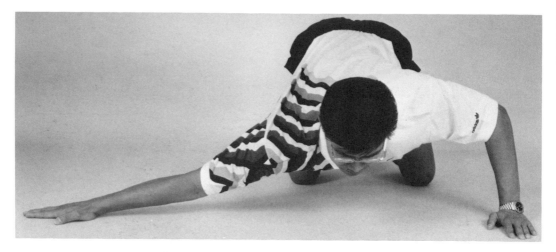

Fig 81   Pectorals and deltoids.

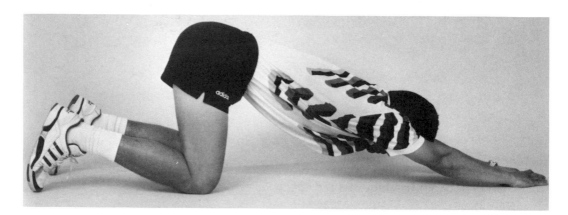

Fig 82   Shoulders.

PECTORAL AND DELTOID STRETCH
(Fig 81)
While kneeling on all fours on a padded surface, take one arm to the side, in line with the shoulder. Without hyperextending the elbow, gently lower the shoulder to the floor. Take care not to arch or twist the back. Repeat on the other side.

SHOULDER STRETCH
(Fig 82)
Kneeling with the hips directly over the knees, and taking care not to arch the back, cross the thumbs and place the hands on the floor in a forward position. Now lower the chest and face to the floor.

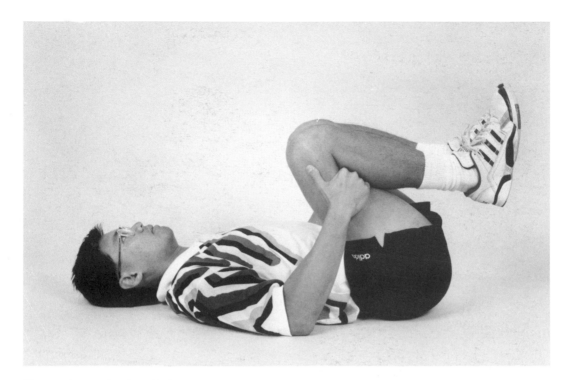

Fig 83   Lower back and gluteals.

LOWER-BACK AND GLUTEAL STRETCH
(Fig 83)
Lie flat on the back with the knees drawn into the chest. Hold the legs behind the knees so as not to flex them excessively, and relax in this position. This is also an excellent stretch for easing tension in the spine.

HAMSTRING STRETCH
(Fig 84)
Lie on the back with one leg straight and the other bent. The straight leg is eased into the chest. It may be necessary to bend the knee slightly as shown, but if possible, keep it straight. Instead of bending the knee a great deal, use a towel as shown in figs 91 or 92 in the next section.

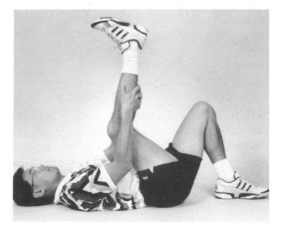

Fig 84   Hamstrings.

83

STRETCHING FOR TEAM GAMES

HIP FLEXOR AND RHOMBOID STRETCH
(Fig 85)
Take a moderate step forwards and lower the rear knee to the floor. A right angle is important on the front knee, as is a straight back to avoid leaning forwards, which reduces the stretch on the psoas major, an important kicking muscle. Link the hands and reach forwards. Repeat and change legs.

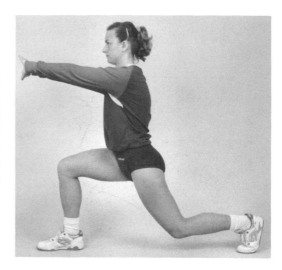

Fig 85   Hip flexors and rhomboids.

STANDING HAMSTRING STRETCH
(Fig 86)
When stretching outdoors it is impractical to lie on the floor, therefore the standing hamstring stretch is very useful. Stretch one leg at a time by taking a leg forwards, bending the rear leg, and placing the hands on it. This supports the spine. By leaning forwards and tilting the pelvis so that the bottom moves down and back, the top of the pelvis moves forwards. A stretch is felt in the hamstrings of the straight leg. Repeat on the other side.

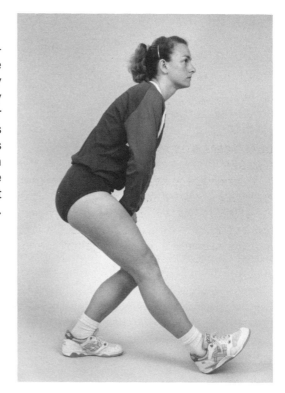

Fig 86   Standing hamstring stretch.

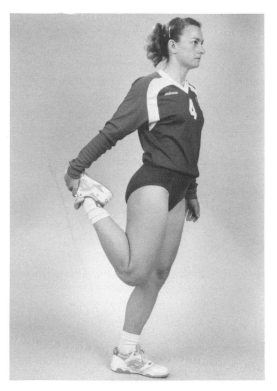

Fig 87   Quadriceps.

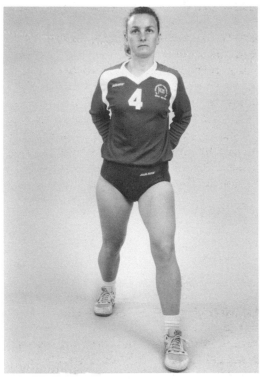

Fig 88   Gastrocnemius and pectorals.

QUADRICEPS STRETCH
(Fig 87)
It is important to keep the knees together and push the hips forwards in this stretch. The body should remain upright, but the spine must not be arched. If it is hard to balance, then lean against a wall.

GASTROCNEMIUS AND PECTORAL STRETCH
(Fig 88)
With a good base, take a step back, push the rear heel into the floor and ensure the foot points forwards. Bend the front knee and feel the calf stretch. At the same time, link the hands behind the back and pull the shoulder blades together to stretch the chest.

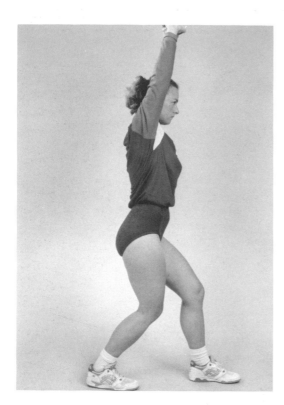

Fig 89 Shoulders and lower calves.

SHOULDER AND LOWER-CALF STRETCH
(Fig 89)
As in fig 88, but bend the rear leg and push the knee down to the ground. At the same time raise the arms above the head, link the thumbs and press the arms back. Repeat and change legs.

ADDUCTOR AND QUADRATUS LUMBORUM STRETCH
(Fig 90)
Take a side lunge position, ensuring that the knee of the bent leg is over the toe, and that the foot of the straight leg does not roll inwards. Rest one arm on the thigh of the bent leg, reach up with the opposite hand, and lean over as shown. Repeat on the other side.

Fig 90 Adductors and quadratus lumborum.

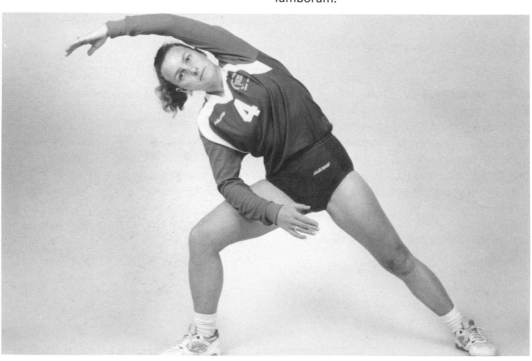

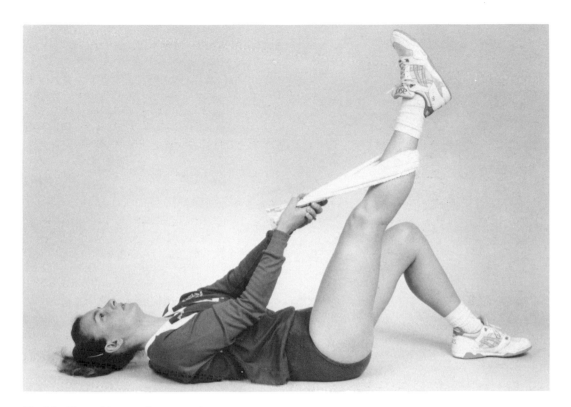

Fig 91   Towel hamstring stretch.

TOWEL HAMSTRING STRETCH
(Fig 91)
Lie with a flat back, one leg bent, and the other as straight as possible without causing pain. Wrap a towel around the calf and ease the leg towards the chest. Try to relax and not to force this position. Repeat on the other side.

TOWEL HAMSTRING STRETCH VARIATION
(Fig 92)
Some people will feel more comfortable in this position. However, it is important to lean forwards from the hips, and not the spine, to gain maximum benefit.

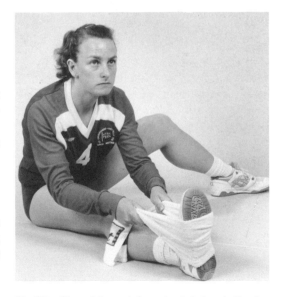

Fig 92   Towel hamstring stretch (variation).

87

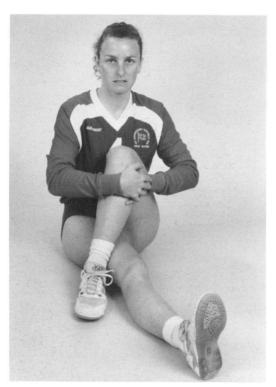

Fig 93   Abductors.

STRETCHES FOR RUNNING/JUMPING ACTIVITIES

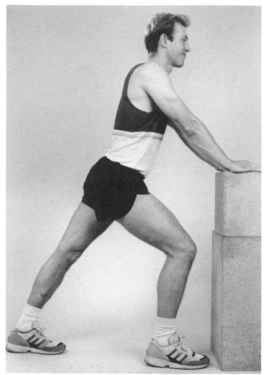

Fig 94   Supported gastrocnemius.

ABDUCTOR STRETCH
(Fig 93)
Sit with one bent leg lifted across one straight leg, hold the outside of the knee and ease the leg in towards and across the chest. Repeat on the other side.

SUPPORTED GASTROCNEMIUS STRETCH
(Fig 94)
Lean against a stable chair or wall so that one leg can be taken back and the heel of that leg pushed into the ground. The front knee should be bent, and the weight moved towards the wall. Repeat on the other leg.

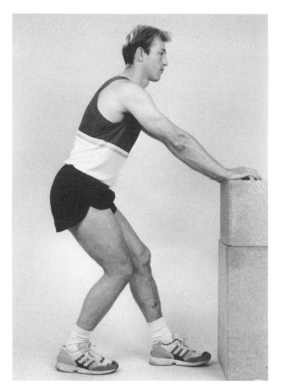

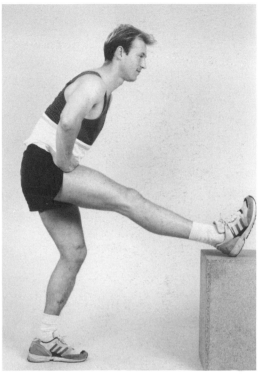

Fig 95   Supported lower calves.

Fig 96   Supported hamstrings.

SUPPORTED LOWER-CALF STRETCH
(Fig 95)
As in fig 94 except the rear leg is bent.
The action is to push the knee downwards and adopt a slight sitting position
as shown. This is a very important
stretch, especially for runners, as this
area can become very tight. Repeat on
the other side.

SUPPORTED HAMSTRING STRETCH
(Fig 96)
Place one foot on a block or low wall and
bend the other leg slightly to improve
balance. With the hands placed on the
hips to support the spine, lean the body
forwards to feel the stretch. It is
important that the lean comes from the
hips and not from the spine. Repeat on
the other side.

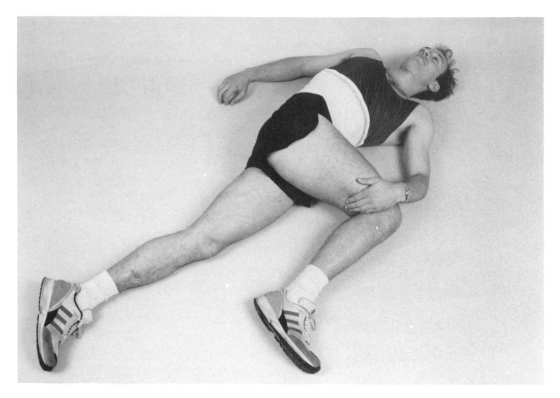

Fig 97   Abductors and iliotibial band.

LYING ABDUCTOR AND ILIOTIBIAL BAND STRETCH
(Fig 97)
While lying on the back, bend one leg and take it across the other leg, which is straight. Using the hand, add a little pressure to increase the stretch as shown.

LYING SPINAL STRETCH
(Fig 98)
Spread the arms for balance, as shown, and move the legs slowly to one side, flexing at the knees and hips. It is important to relax in this position and to repeat on the other side.

LYING QUADRICEP STRETCH
(Fig 99)
Lie with the head supported as shown, the lower leg slightly bent, and the upper leg flexed at the knee. Hold the ankle and push the hip forwards. Repeat on the other side.

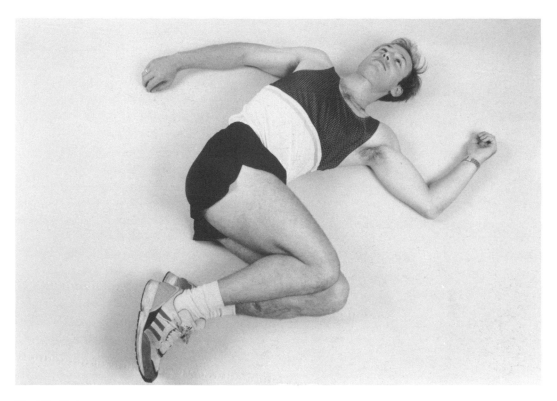

Fig 98   Spine.

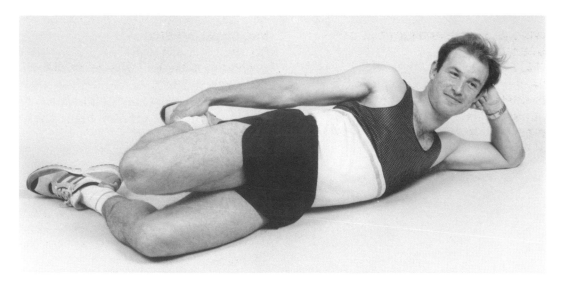

Fig 99   Quadriceps.

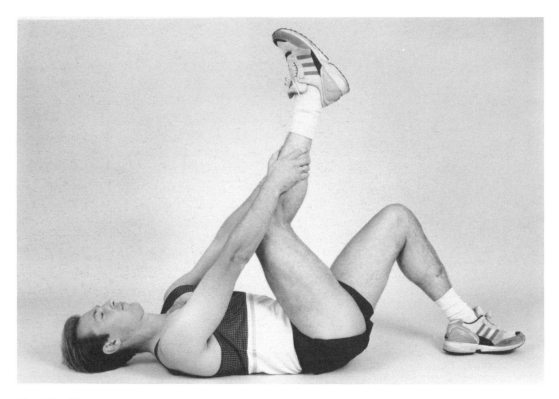

Fig 100   Hamstrings.

LYING HAMSTRING STRETCH
(Fig 100)
While lying on the back with one leg bent, ease the other leg in towards the chest. If this is difficult, try the towel version indicated in fig 91 in the 'Team Games' section.

LOWER AND UPPER BACK STRETCH
(Fig 101)
Sit with the legs bent and parallel. Place the hands on the floor behind the back, and push the weight gently forwards. At the same time ease the chin to the chest.

LOWER BACK AND GLUTEAL STRETCH
(Fig 102)
Hold behind the knees, pulling the legs into the chest, while lying on the back to ease the pressure on the spine. This is a very relaxing recovery stretch.

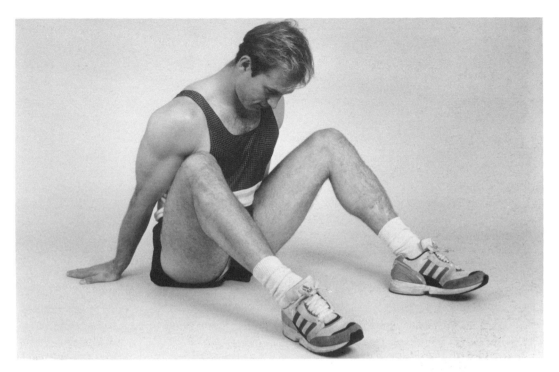

Fig 101   Lower and upper back.

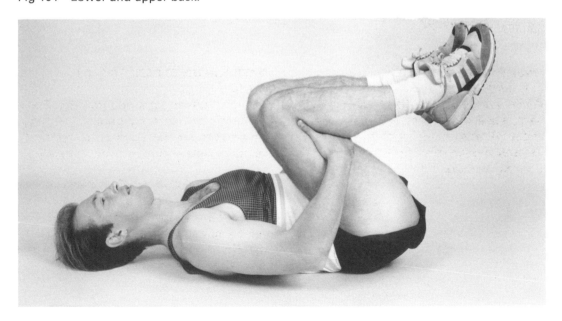

Fig 102   Lower back and gluteals.

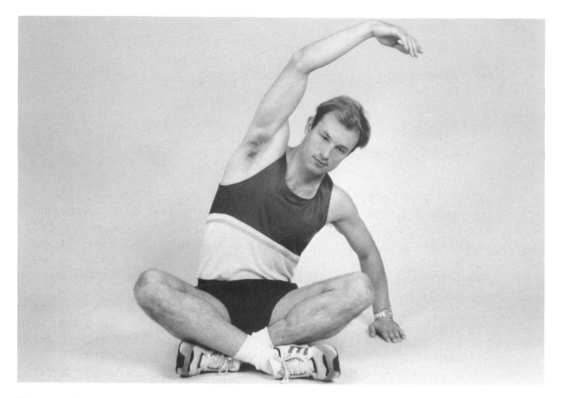

Fig 103   Quadratus lumborum.

QUADRATUS LUMBORUM STRETCH
(Fig 103)
While sitting with crossed (or parallel) legs, place one hand on the floor, stretch up with the other arm and reach over the head. Pull the abdominals in and take care not to allow the back to sag.

7

Designing a Training Programme

It appears clear that, unless an individual is one of a small minority who is over-flexible or *hyper-flexible*, then the more stretching we can do the better. Those individuals who are very flexible will need to monitor their ROM and keep a sensible balance between strength and flexibility in all the joint complexes.

For those with less than perfect flexibility, as much stretching as possible should be included in the training programme, provided the safe techniques that have been indicated in this book are followed. How much flexibility training there is in any one programme will to a large extent become a function of the time available. Traditionally, flexibility training has always been the last item on the list and consequently neglected by many people. I would suggest that this is a mistake and that athletes, as well as fitness-conscious individuals, should look for ways of committing themselves to a flexibility training regime.

With this in mind, what follows are three examples of a *typical* training week at different times of the year, for three selected activities. They are intended to show how flexibility training can be integrated into an individual's programme.

As a starting point, I would encourage everyone to begin to include a thorough warm-up into their programme whenever they begin to exercise, be it for a practice, a game, a competition, or indeed, for a flexibility training session. Short-hold stretches should be included as part of this warm-up. Similarly, at the end of an exercise session, the same stretches can be performed again as part of a cool-down, preferably supplemented by long-hold stretches.

If this practice were to be adopted, it would represent a major step forwards in an individual's active lifestyle and training programme. In addition, the use of partner stretches and PNF variations can be incorporated where appropriate, as indicated in the programmes below.

Once flexibility training becomes part of your regular routine, you will see it as a natural feature and one which you will not want to leave out. You may find that there are times of the year when you have more time to spend on stretching and you should take full advantage of this. Long winter evenings are excellent for devoting time to stretching in the warmth of your own home. Not only is this very relaxing, but it is very rewarding as well.

WINTER PROGRAMME FOR AN ÉLITE SWIMMER

Day	A.M.	P.M.	Eve.
Monday	Endurance maintenance	Weight training free weights Partner stretches (not PNF)	Endurance threshold
Tuesday	Endurance recovery, plus technique		Anaerobic training
Wednesday	Endurance recovery, plus technique	Circuit training plus PNF stretching as a group	
Thursday			Endurance threshold
Friday	Endurance recovery, plus technique		Endurance overload, plus power work
Saturday	Endurance maintenance, plus starts and turns	Machine weights PNF stretches	
Sunday			Specific stretches as an individual

Key:

Endurance recovery: low intensity, for example 6,000m, mixed strokes including kicking and pulling. Long intervals.

Endurance maintenance: medium intensity, for example 6,000m, mixed strokes including kicking and pulling. Medium/long intervals.

Endurance threshold: high intensity, for example 5,000m, front crawl, medium intervals, short recovery.

Endurance overload: very high intensity, for example 4,500m, main stroke, medium intervals, medium recovery.

Anaerobic training: very high intensity, for example 3,500m, main stroke, short intervals, long recovery. Distances refer to the total length of the session including warm-up and cool-down.

PROGRAMME FOR A COUNTY-STANDARD HOCKEY PLAYER DURING THE MAIN SEASON

Day	A.M.	P.M.	Eve.
Monday	H1 personal session		Specific stretches
Tuesday			Game
Wednesday			
Thursday	Partner stretching		Squad session
Friday	H2 personal session		
Saturday		Game	PNF stretching
Sunday			Specific stretches

Key:

H1 personal session: high intensity, short duration, for example speed work.
Squad session: for example maintenance fitness, plus teamwork and set plays, long duration.
H2 personal session: moderate intensity, moderate duration, for example, circuit training.

Players should use short-hold stretches before and after all the above sessions and before and after the games. Where possible short- and long-hold stretches should be included in the cool-downs, with particular emphasis on the 'Team Game' stretches in Chapter 6. Specific flexibility sessions should take approximately 30 minutes to complete.

SUMMER PROGRAMME FOR A COMMITTED RECREATIONAL DISTANCE RUNNER

Day	A.M.	P.M.	Eve.
Monday	Run 1 or rest		Specific stretches
Tuesday			Interval training
Wednesday	Run 2		Weight training
Thursday		Fartlek run	
Friday	Run 3		
Saturday			Specific stretches
Sunday		10km (6 mile) road race	Partner stretches

Key:

Run 1: long, easy run, 1 – 1¼ hours.
Run 2: short, easy run, 30 – 40 minutes.
Run 3: short, easy run, striding towards the end, 30 minutes.
Interval training: hard effort, for example, four times 1,000m with 2 minutes recovery.
Fartlek run: speed play in a wood or a park.
Weight training: very light repetitions.

Runners should stretch before and after all sessions as part of the warming-up and cooling-down procedures, as well as during the specific sessions indicated. Specific sessions should take approximately 30 minutes to complete.

8

Research into Flexibility

Having considered in some detail in earlier chapters the theoretical and practical implications of flexibility training, both for athletes and fitness-conscious individuals, this section concentrates on some of the readily available research findings on flexibility. These form the basis for approaching the development of ROM in a safe, effective and enjoyable way.

Where someone's name is indicated, for example, Hardy (1986) or Cornelius (1988), it indicates that the statement refers to this person's work. A full bibliography for these works can be found in the 'Further Reading' section for the interested reader to follow up.

The research on flexibility, stretching and related areas of interest such as joints, bones, muscles and tendon attachments, has not covered the issue of flexibility training to any great extent. It is generally believed to be quite difficult to standardize procedures in this area because of the multitude of factors that might influence the outcome. These factors include body temperature, room temperature, time of day, age and gender of the individual, and training status, both on the day and more generally. However, there have been some useful studies, and where I refer to them I will give a full reference for them under 'Further Reading'.

Flexibility, as we have seen, has been described as the range of motion (ROM) possible in a joint or group of joints, where the ROM is specific to each joint (Cornelius and Craft-Hamm, 1988). Because of this specificity, a thorough knowledge of the action potential of joints and the musculature is most important, hence the detailed approach this text has taken. With this knowledge, it is possible to devise more accurately programmes to affect specific body parts in a way that is safe and effective for the type of work being performed.

BIOPHYSICAL FACTORS

The structure of the joint is important for determining the normal range of movement, but as Corbin et al (1990) point out, other factors are even more vital for determining flexibility: that is, muscles, ligaments and, to a lesser extent, tendons. As Wright and Johns (1962) show clearly, 47 per cent of the restriction to movement is caused by the joint shape, which is effectively unchangeable. What can be changed, however, are the 'soft' tissue elements. It is the elasticity in these structures that is vital to flexibility, and work on improving ROM will, in Hartley O'Brien's (1983) terms, 'provide greater mechanical efficiency, improve aesthetic appeal and possibly play a role in injury prevention'.

99

Since the only way to improve flexibility is through stretching, the athlete must have a thorough knowledge of the different types of stretch available and how to execute them safely.

There are two types of flexibility methods studied in the literature, namely static and dynamic. Static flexibility training can be further sub-divided into active and passive movements. Corbin (1980) defines static stretching as 'slow, sustained stretching exercises that place a muscle in a lengthened position and hold that position for a few seconds'. Dynamic flexibility he defines as 'a type of stretching exercise involving bouncing or jerking to gain momentum in the body to enhance over-stretching'.

Active stretches are those that use unassisted movements, which requires strength and muscular effort of the agonist muscle (prime mover). Passive movements are accomplished through the use of an external force such as that provided by a partner, gravity or momentum. All other methods of stretching, such as proprioceptive neuromuscular facilitation (PNF), or contract-relax with agonist contraction (CRAC) are variations of these. However, it is important for the athlete to be aware of the current literature on these methods to ascertain which are the most beneficial, or the most appropriate, in a given sport or training session.

Although gymnasts, aerobic championship performers or skaters may use many ballistic movements in their routines, the majority of experts would not recommend that ballistic stretching be carried out to simulate these. Etnyre and Lee (1987) state that ballistic stretching has fallen into disfavour because of the possibility that injury may result from the abrupt stretch. Since ballistic stretching is believed to be more traumatic to the muscle, static stretching is generally recommended by authors of currently popular stretching programmes.

However, Hardy and Jones (1986) suggest that dynamic flexibility is probably more important in speed events, like, perhaps, championship aerobics, some games or athletic activities. It must be remembered, though, that this does not necessarily mean that ballistic movements are the optimum method for acquiring flexibility, merely that they are a part of certain sports.

Many competitors will use a combination of both active and passive movements in their routines; for example, a split leap uses a great deal of flexibility, and requires very strong agonists in order to achieve the correct position, whereas the box splits on the floor is a passive position. Kicking and sprinting are extremely dynamic actions, as are hurdling and pole vaulting. There is a dichotomy in the literature that has not been conclusively resolved, about whether these actions should be used to develop flexibility in their own right, or used more specifically in training that is supplemented by less aggressive means of stretching.

Since an increase in muscle suppleness in the antagonist is of little use unless accompanied by an increase in the muscular strength of the agonist, it would seem that flexibility training using contraction of the agonists would be of particular benefit. Hartley O'Brien (1980) reasoned that as active flexibility was the 'maximum unassisted range of movement', it should be possible to increase

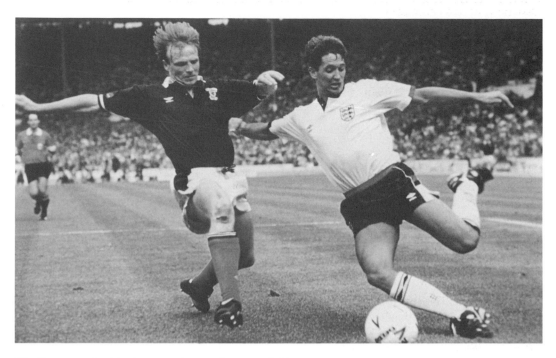

Hip flexor and adductor suppleness is essential in soccer.

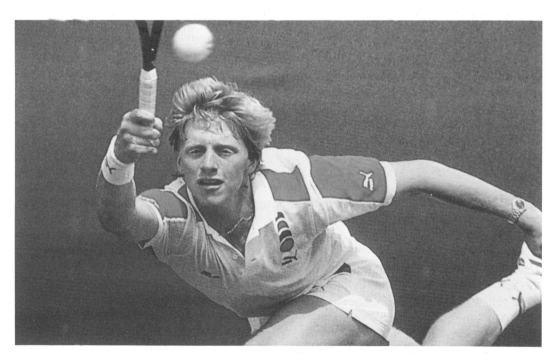

Lunging and reaching: two key aspects of the game of tennis.

this by either decreasing the resistance of the antagonist, or increasing the strength of the agonist. This is the basis of PNF techniques, especially the CRAC method.

Hardy (1985) conducted experiments that agreed with Hartley O'Brien's hypothesis that 'active flexibility is best increased by utilising techniques which maximise strength gains in the agonists and relaxation in the antagonists', as shown in methods such as PNF stretching. Clearly this is an important consideration when preparing for speed events where agility and speed of movement are essential. Perhaps it is less so, however, for a member of the general public who wants simply to improve overall fitness and health, or for some performers with less specific needs. The distinction is an important one.

Another major area of vital knowledge for the athlete in relation to flexibility, concerns the connective tissues of the body. Wright and Johns (1962) indicate that 41 per cent of the resistance to ROM comes from the muscle and its fascia, and a further 10 per cent is attributable to the tendon. I have shown how connective tissues are made up of elastic and viscous properties. Viscosity is mainly attributable to collagen, which has a triple-helix arrangement of fibres that form cross-linkages with glyco-aminoglycans extracellularly in the connective tissues (Booth, 1975). This makes collagen incredibly strong but not very elastic. Fibroblasts (another type of connective tissue) similarly offer a good deal of resistance to movement; but elastin, in contrast, is an elastic tissue.

The important point is that all connective tissues have some degree of elasticity which, as Corbin and Noble (1980) indicate, is affected by temperature. If warmed, muscles and connective tissues will become more responsive to stretch. Mobility exercises (movements in the inner and middle range of a joint) will help increase muscle temperature prior to stretching. Martin et al (1975) indicate that 'the increased heat production associated with muscular exercise leads to a rapid temperature rise in the working muscles and a more gradual temperature rise in the body core. Higher temperatures during exercise reduce viscosity (resistance) and increase rate of nerve conduction.' Also, 'the dissociation of oxygen from haemoglobin is more complete at a higher muscle temperature, thus enhancing oxygen supply during work.'

Sapega et al (1981) also recommend a thorough warm-up, and state that stretching should not be done at the beginning of a warm-up routine when tissue temperature is very low: 'all of the data reviewed would indicate that cold muscles and tendons are less "stretchable" and more vulnerable to accidental injury through over-zealous stretching.' Sapega points out that at 104°F (40°C) 'a thermal transition occurs, which significantly enhances the viscous-stress relaxation of collagenous tissue, allowing greater plastic deformation when it is stretched.' In simple terms this means that muscle and connective tissue respond better when warm, especially when this temperature is above a certain critical level (104°F/40°C).

However, one further important point mentioned in Sapega's (1981) paper is that some degree of mechanical weakening may take place when connective tissue structures are permanently elongated; the amount of weakening depends on the way in which the tissue is stretched as well as how much it is stretched. It is worth noting, in the light of my earlier comments on static and ballistic stretching, that it is ballistic stretching that produces maximum structural weakening, and static stretching that produces the least. This provides us with a major piece of evidence, that static techniques are safer. In addition, the long-hold static stretch appears to be most effective for stretching connective tissue, which forms the largest area of changeable resistance (41 per cent) for the exercising individual. PNF techniques give further improvements.

NEUROLOGICAL FACTORS

More important evidence on this subject is unearthed when one considers the neurological implications of flexibility training, rather than the biophysical factors considered so far. The two main neurological concerns pertain to the myotatic stretch reflex and the golgi-tendon organ reflex.

As I have shown, the myotatic reflex occurs in every muscle when it is being stretched, and is a response to prevent damage to the muscle. When a muscle is stretched too quickly an impulse is sent to cause contraction in that muscle. Since stretching will now work in opposition to contraction, the suggestion is that possible damage to the muscle may occur in the form of microscopic tearing. The important point is that the magnitude of the stretch reflex is proportional to the speed of movement (Alter, 1988): that is, the faster the movement, the greater the stretch reflex response, and the greater the risk of damage to the muscle tissues.

This, of course, lends more support to the argument for the using of static stretching techniques, as ballistic movements produce stretch reflexes repeatedly. The harder the bounce, the worse it is for the muscle. When stretches are held, whatever initial contraction there has been in the muscle will dissipate; this desensitization of the stretch reflex occurs in the first few seconds (Alter 1988). Following this, collagen creeping occurs to allow greater movement (relaxation) and to facilitate relatively permanent deformation of the collagen. Muscle creeping is thought to occur next, although, unlike collagen, muscle will return to its normal length when the stretch is removed because it is an elastic tissue.

The major limiting factor to flexibility, as Sapega's (1981) work shows, is the viscous, connective tissue surrounding muscle and in tendons. The longer the stretches are held, and the warmer the tissue, the better will be the results. De Vries (1961) had success with a hold of 2 minutes, whereas Beaulieu (1981) and Moore and Hutton (1970) suggest 30–60 seconds as useful parameters. In all cases, repeating stretches is thought to be important, as is stretching on a regular daily basis.

The second neurological response relates to the golgi-tendon organ reflex (GTO). GTOs respond to and monitor the tension in the muscle spindles, but are themselves situated at the junction of the muscle and tendon. If tension in a muscle becomes great enough to stimulate the GTOs, they send a warning message which, in turn, will produce a reflex relaxation in the tensioned

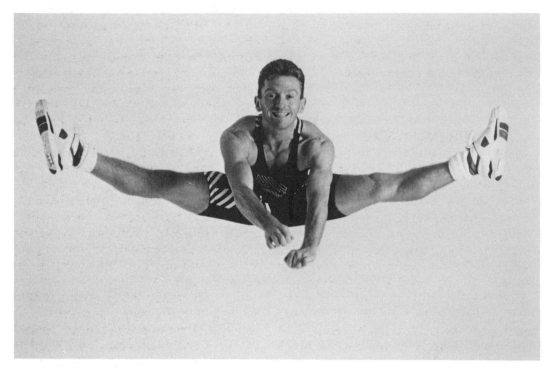

And he smiles as well! An excellent example of dynamic flexibility in a split leap.

muscle. The GTOs are therefore protective mechanisms (McAtee, 1993). However, the high threshold level required to make the GTOs respond means that it takes a strong tension for them to come into play, and such tension is difficult to achieve through stretching. Tension through contraction, however, is much easier to achieve and hence the contract-relax, CRAC and PNF techniques are preferable in this respect.

The isometric contraction common to both methods causes tension to develop in the muscle, stimulating the GTOs. The debate in scientific literature had tended to focus on the optimum duration of this contraction. Cornelius and Hinson (1980) found no significant difference in improved ROM between isometric contractions held for 3 as opposed to 6 seconds; Hardy (1985) found a positive linear relationship between improved ROM and duration of contraction, that is, the longer the contraction the greater the response. More recently, Nelson and Cornelius (1991) used 3-, 6- and 10-second contractions and, again, found no significant difference as far as ROM was concerned.

The implication of this research might be that, given the fact that long-duration isometric contractions elevate blood pressure significantly, the 3–10-second parameter can safely be used with no detrimental side-effects. This applies both to contract-relax techniques and CRAC techniques; in the latter the end position is also held by the performer using an isometric contraction of the agonist.

INJURY PREVENTION

The final area of interest concerns the issue of injury prevention. The main thrust of the argument for flexibility training in this regard is that, through having a greater range of movement, there is more scope for a muscle to lengthen in the event of a stretch at speed. Consequently, when a muscle is stretched, but not as far as its ultimate range, there is less chance of it being damaged. As Corbin (1989) puts it, 'A shortened muscle is apparently much more likely to exceed its normal range of extensibility than one which has been lengthened through training'.

A reasonable level of flexibility is also desirable for good health. Many back problems are attributable to weak or unsupple muscles. Weak abdominals are another example of the former, and tight hamstrings or hip flexors of the latter.

Most authorities agree that stretching has a role to play in the prevention of injury but, in fact, there is currently a dearth of evidence. Much of it is speculative or applied from other areas of sports science. One interesting hypothesis, however, is that post-exercise stretching will prevent the onset of muscle soreness in the days to follow. Although this is commonly believed among athletes, there is little evidence to support it. De Vries (1961) was one of the first to suggest that stretching does help; however, more recently Buroker and Schwane (1989) could not agree and failed to find any evidence for static stretching as a means of relief from either acute or chronic muscle soreness. If overload has been so severe as to cause muscle damage, it appears unlikely that stretching, or anything else for that matter, could prevent the inevitable soreness.

I have reviewed a large amount of the available literature on the areas that are perhaps of most interest to the personal trainer or coach who may have to advise the 'average' sedentary individual, the exercise enthusiast, or the élite performer in a sport. Static stretching in its many forms – personal, partner, PNF, CRAC – gains most favour in terms of safety and effectiveness, while ballistic stretching is regarded as very high risk and often ineffective as far as the connective tissues are concerned. As connective tissue appears to be the most significant changeable factor, it seems that static stretching of warm tissue should be the most beneficial option in the long term.

9
Summary

It is hoped that, by following the rational and programme prescription indicated in this book, the athlete or interested participant will get much enjoyment and benefit from stretching. Unsafe stretching as characterized by poor technique or high risk practices has been avoided because I feel the cost outweighs the potential benefit. The reader can feel sure, therefore, that the stretches will be beneficial in the daily regime and will enhance performance and physical well-being.

Stretching can be performed at any time of day, and as often as required; unlike some other forms of training, stretching will not damage the tissues of the body, so it will not need time to repair itself after a stretching session. Furthermore, it seems to be clear that incorporating stretching in an individual's daily routine will help combat the relentless ageing process.

I would therefore encourage everyone to stretch regularly, and to enjoy the positive feelings associated with feeling good about the supple body that is being created.

Glossary

Afferent message A message that is sent from the muscle to the brain.

Agonist The main muscle responsible for a joint movement, also called the prime mover.

Antagonist The muscle that opposes the action of the agonist, allowing joint movement.

Anterior To the front of the body.

Articular surface The surface of a bone that comes together with another bone to form a joint.

Ballistic A dynamic action involving speed of movement.

Cartilage Firm gristly tissue, which aids shock absorption in a joint.

Cobra An extreme spinal stretch, which places great strain on the lumbar and cervical vertebrae.

Collagen A protein connective tissue, which is very strong but not very elastic.

Connective tissue The general term for tissue that connects muscle to bone or muscle fibres to other muscle fibres.

Coracoid process The small, bony protrusion in the front of the shoulder, close to the ball-and-socket joint.

Clavicular Referring to the clavicle, or a portion of the clavicle (collar bone).

CRAC Contraction, relaxation, agonist contraction (a form of PNF stretching).

Cruciate Refers to the ligaments that cross the knee to the front and rear, hence anterior and posterior cruciate ligaments.

Deltoid The shoulder muscle responsible mainly for abduction and which assists in other movements such as flexion and extension.

Efferent Message A message that is sent from the brain to the muscles.

Elastic A protein connective tissue with elastic properties.

Extensor A muscle responsible for extending a joint.

Fibroblast A form of loose connective tissue.

Flexibility Range of movement.

Flexor A muscle responsible for flexing a joint.

Golgi-Tendon Organs Protective receptors based at the junction of the muscle and tendon.

Hyperextension A movement that goes beyond the normal range of extension.

Hyperflexion A tightly flexed position, or deep flexion.

Intercostals The muscles between the ribs that assist in supporting the rib cage.

107

Isometric A form of muscle contraction that produces tension but does not involve movement.

Ligament A structure that connects bone to bone in joints.

Lumbar The lowest five vertebrae of the spine situated above the sacrum.

Lymph Glands that are similar to veins and convey the passage of lymph fluid, a blood-like substance without red corpuscles.

Mobility Movement in a joint, especially in inner and middle ranges; this term is sometimes used synonymously with flexibility.

Muscle Fibres Fibres that are arranged in bundles making up the muscle as a whole.

Myofibrils Small fibres that make up muscle fibres.

Muscle Spindles Nerve endings that allow the muscle to be stimulated.

Myotatic Stretch Reflex A protective mechanism that responds when the muscle is quickly stretched.

Over-Stretching A technique that stretches tissues beyond their normal range.

Patella The knee-cap.

Plough An exercise involving extreme flexion of the spine, which is capable of straining the neck badly.

PNF Proprioceptive neuromuscular facilitation – an advanced stretching technique.

Posterior To the rear of the body.

Proprioceptors Receptors that detect where the limb is in relation to other limbs or in general space.

Reciprocal Innervation A technical term explaining that as one muscle contracts, its opposite relaxes.

Rhomboid A muscle situated between the shoulder blades.

Sarcomere The functional, contractile part of the myofibril.

Somatotype A person's genetic body type which indicates particular characteristics of muscularity, fatness or leanness.

Suppleness Stretchability of muscle and connective tissue.

Synovial Fluid A joint lubricant that promotes the smooth running of the joint surfaces.

Synovial Joint A freely movable joint in the body. All synovial joints have a similar structure.

Tendon A structure that connects muscle to bone.

Viscosity Resistance to stretch.

Further Reading

Alter, M.J., *The Science of Stretching*, Human Kinetics, Illinois (1989)

Beaulieu, J.E., 'Developing a stretching programme', *Physician and Sports Medicine*, 9 (11), 1981, pp. 59 – 69

Booth, F.W. and Gould, E.W., 'Effects of training and disuse on connective tissue', *Exercise and Sports Science Review*, 3, 1975, pp. 83 – 112

Buroker, M.R. and Schwane, J.A., 'Does post-exercise static stretching alleviate delayed muscle soreness?', *Physician and Sports Medicine*, 17 (6), 1989, pp. 65 – 83

Corbin, C.V. and Noble, L., 'Flexibility: a major component of physical fitness', *Journal of Physical Education and Recreation'* 51 (6), 1980, pp. 23 – 4 and 57 – 60

Cornelius, W.L. and Craft-Hamm, K., 'Proprioceptive Neuromuscular Facilitation flexibility techniques: acute effects on arterial blood pressure', *Physician and Sports Medicine*, 16 (4), 1988, pp. 152 – 61

Cornelius, W.L. and Hinson, M.M., 'The relationship between isometric contraction of hip extensors and subsequent flexibility in males', *Journal of Sports Medicine and Physical Fitness*, 20, 1980, 75 – 80

De Vries, H.A., 'Prevention of muscular distress after exercise', *Research Quarterly*, 32, 1961, pp. 177 – 185

Etnyre, B.R. and Abraham, L.D., 'Antagonist muscle activity during stretching: a paradox reassessed', *Medical Science and Sports Exercise*, 20 (3), 1988, pp. 285 – 9

Etnyre, B.R. and Lee, E.J., 'Comments on PNF stretching techniques', *Research Quarterly*, 58, 1986, pp. 1 – 5

Hardy, L., 'Improving active range of hip flexion', *Research Quarterly*, 56 (2), 1985, pp. 111 – 14

Hardy, L. and Jones, D., 'Dynamic flexibility and proprioceptive neuro-muscular facilitation', *Research Quarterly*, 57, 1986, pp. 105 – 53

Hartley O'Brien, S.J., 'Six mobilisation exercises for active range of hip flexion', *Research Quarterly*, 51 (4), 1980, pp. 625 – 35

McAtee, R.E., *Facilitated Stretching*, Human Kinetics, Illinois (1993)

Martin, B.J. *et al*, 'Effect of warm up on metabolic response to strenuous exercise', *Medicine, Sport and Exercise*, 7 (2), 1975, pp. 146 – 9

Moore, M. and Hutton, R.S., 'Electromyographic investigation of muscle stretching techniques', *Medicine, Science, Sport and Exercise*, 12 (5), 1989, pp. 322 – 9

Nelson, J.K. *et al*, 'Physical characteristics, hip flexibility and arm strength of female gymnasts classified by intensity of training across age', *Journal of Sports, Medicine and Physical Fitness*, 23 (1), 1983, pp. 95 – 100

Nelson, K.C. and Cornelius, W.L., 'The relationship between isometric contraction durations and improvement in shoulder joint ROM', *Journal of Sports, Medicine and Physical Fitness*, 31 (3), 1991, pp. 385 – 88

Sapega, A.A. *et al,* 'Biophysical factors in range of motion exercise', *Physician and Sports Medicine* 9 (12), 1981, pp. 57 – 65

Wright, V. and Johns, R.J., 'Relative importance of various tissues in joint stiffness', *Journal of Applied Physiology,* 17 (5), 1962, pp. 824 – 8

Index